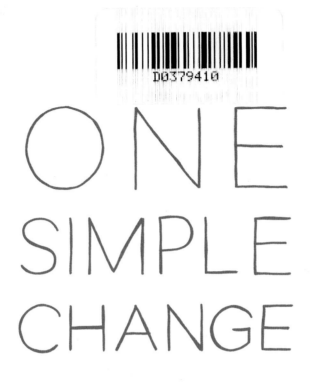

ONE SIMPLE CHANGE

SURPRISINGLY EASY WAYS *to*
TRANSFORM YOUR LIFE

—— Winnie Abramson, ND ——

CHRONICLE BOOKS
SAN FRANCISCO

Library of Congress Cataloging-in-Publication Data:

Abramson, Winnie.
 One simple change : surprisingly easy ways to transform your life /
Winnie Abramson.
   pages cm
 ISBN 978-1-4521-1957-1
1. Nutrition. 2. Health—Nutritional aspects. 3. Holistic medicine—
Popular works. 4. Vegetarianism—Popular works. I. Title.

 RA784.A26 2013
 613.2—dc23

                         2013002292

Manufactured in China

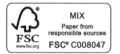

Designed by Hillary Caudle
Icons designed by Hillary Caudle and Sean McCormick

10 9 8 7 6 5 4 3 2 1

Chronicle Books LLC
680 Second Street
San Francisco, California 94107
www.chroniclebooks.com

CONTENTS

INTRODUCTION

WHEN I WAS SIXTEEN, I decided to lose 5 lb/2.3 kg. I was an active teen on the thin side of normal, but all my friends were dieting, so I figured I might as well join them. It was the eighties and the low-fat dieting craze was in full swing. I jumped on the bandwagon and waited for the weight to melt away.

It didn't, but I kept dieting anyway. I'd grown up on the fabulous butter- and cream-laden fare my dad prepared in the kitchen of my family's four-star restaurant The Quilted Giraffe, but magazine articles on weight loss and health said these delicacies could no longer pass through my lips. I became convinced that if low fat was good, then no fat must be better; I also proclaimed myself a vegetarian.

The list of things I would eat got smaller and smaller. I subsisted mainly on salads and cooked vegetables doused with vinegar, cottage cheese, and bagels—and I was constantly hungry. I thought about sweets nearly all the time, and I drank diet sodas and downed large servings of frozen yogurt to quell the cravings.

I told myself the diet was only temporary; I'd go off it as soon as I morphed into superskinny Winnie. But when the needle on my scale finally began to move, it went in the wrong direction. I was horrified that I was gaining weight, but I never once questioned the diet; in fact, I went away to college and kept on dieting for another four years.

Despite rigidly controlling my calorie intake and running or taking aerobics classes nearly every day, I weighed about 15 lb/6.8 kg more than I wanted to (10 lb/4.5 kg more than when I had first started dieting) by the time graduation rolled around. At that point, I was also tired all day long and extremely depressed; my face was covered with pimples; and my menstrual cycle had all but disappeared. I felt perfectly awful, yet I still stubbornly believed my diet was perfect.

I visited one doctor after another in the hopes that someone would discover what was wrong with me. I was referred to counselors to talk about the depression, and I was given prescriptions for antibiotics to make the acne go away. I was given no explanation for why I was always so exhausted.

When an endocrinologist diagnosed me with a scary-sounding condition called polycystic ovary syndrome (PCOS) to explain why I so rarely menstruated, my mom suggested we go to a different type of health practitioner for a second opinion—a holistic one. This was the first time in my life that I had heard that term.

Appointments with my new doctor were vastly different from what I was accustomed to: She seemed genuinely interested in getting to the bottom of what was going on with me; she did not look at (or try to provide solutions for) my health issues in isolation; and she did not think I had PCOS. She asked a lot of questions that no doctor had ever asked me before, and she gave me a "diet diary," a way for me to log what I ate for a week. I proudly filled it in, smug in my belief that no one had a better diet than I.

After a slew of blood tests, the nutritionist from my doctor's office called and asked me to come in so we could go over the results. It turned out I had really messed up my body on my so-called healthy diet: I had nutritional deficiencies and numerous food sensitivities. Plus my adrenal glands and my thyroid weren't functioning correctly. The nutritionist impressed upon me the importance of eating very differently from then on if I wanted to get better.

I definitely wanted to get better, but I was very confused. I had been led to believe that a low-fat, vegetarian diet was good. Had I taken that advice too far? Or was it possible that advice was wrong for me (or maybe just plain wrong)? I was skeptical about my nutritionist's recommendations: Avoid wheat, dairy, and white sugar. Load up on whole foods high in vitamins, minerals, and healthy fats. And start eating protein from animal foods again. But I decided to trust her.

What happened over the next few weeks was nothing short of a miracle as far as I was concerned: The weight I'd obsessed over for all those years literally fell away. But maybe even more exciting than the weight loss was how at peace with food I began to feel. I never thought about eating when I wasn't hungry, and my compulsive "need" to exercise completely disappeared. After a few more months, I wasn't depressed anymore, my skin cleared, and my energy level improved. It took longer for my menstrual cycle to return to normal, but that happened eventually, too.

The experience of making myself sick with one diet, and then healing myself with another, had a profound impact on me. I became fascinated with therapeutic eating strategies and other alternative ways to treat illness, and I wanted to learn more about them. I moved across the country to Seattle to study at Bastyr University, one of the only accredited schools in the United States with programs in science-based natural medicine. I graduated with a doctorate in naturopathic medicine in 1998 and have been studying holistic nutrition and all the ingredients of a healthy lifestyle on my own ever since.

In 1999, I started a blog called Healthy Green Kitchen. My intent was to post recipes featuring wholesome, nourishing foods as well as inspiration for "eco-groovy" living. Over the years I've shared hundreds of recipes, along with accounts of my forays into organic gardening, keeping backyard chickens, and beekeeping. At the beginning of 2012, however, I decided to shake things up a little. I went back to my naturopathic roots and embarked on writing a year-long holistic lifestyle series called "One Simple Change."

That series was the inspiration for this book.

Like the blog series, this book is a collection of easy-to-implement yet powerful lifestyle tips that can help you positively transform your health and your life. I shared my diet story earlier so you'd know why I am so passionate about the topic of nutrition, and why, when I was compiling the list of topics I wanted to cover, I felt so strongly that many of them should be related to food. But as big a role as food has played and continues to play in my life, I believe that being truly healthy is about much more. That's why I want you to be sure to pay attention to all the other lifestyle suggestions in this book (and there are many).

One Simple Change takes a holistic approach. It will help you discover how to live in a way that will make you feel great while you decrease your risk for a number of chronic diseases. In addition, making the simple changes suggested in this book will benefit not just your personal health, but the health of our planet, as well.

By design—in order to keep things truly simple—chapters are short and sweet. Though I could have expanded on many concepts, I decided it was best to tell you only what I felt you really needed to know: *why and how you should make the change.* While each chapter can certainly stand on its own, I planned the book with the hope that readers would do the whole thing. There are fifty changes in the book, and I encourage you to make one change per week over the course of a year, with two weeks off whenever you decide to take them; this is why the book is called *One Simple Change*.

While you could rush things and make one change each day for fifty days straight, I don't recommend that. Permanent changes in your habits do not happen overnight. Research shows that new habits are much more likely to last if you take them slow and focus on only one change at a time. Don't feel you have to start this book at the beginning of January, though! Sure, January is a great time to start anew with healthy habits, but so is May. September works, too. And you don't have to start a healthy habit on the first of the month or on a Monday. Anytime you can make a change that will make your life healthier is a good time.

You may be startled by the common-sense nature of some of my tips; know that these are included here because sometimes we ignore the very basics of personal care. I think everyone can benefit from being reminded to pay attention to these. Also, the changes that seem the smallest can have the biggest impact.

I am not necessarily going to be telling you only things you already know, however—this is not a regurgitation of the types of health recommendations that can be found in many other books. In fact, many of my suggestions may surprise you; they will likely fly in the face of the information that you've heard (and trusted) in the past. Be assured, however, that I have spent countless hours sorting through all the confusing and often contradictory health recommendations that are out there in order to bring you the most up-to-date, fact-based, reliable information. The things you will learn in *One Simple Change* honor the wisdom of our ancestors while giving a generous nod to modern science, so you can benefit from both.

I am well aware that many of us are very emotionally invested in our lifestyle patterns and get nervous when our ways are called into question. If that's true for you, I ask that you keep an open mind, even when what I am telling you initially makes you uncomfortable. In many ways *One Simple Change* is about suspending preconceived notions, about accepting that what you thought you knew about how to be healthy isn't necessarily correct. Change can be hard—there's no doubt about that—but change is what this book is about.

You don't need a doctor's approval to do anything in *One Simple Change*; the focus is on lifestyle adjustment, dietary transformation, and attitude overhaul, so there's no medical clearance required. That said, if you're an extremely sedentary person, it's always a good idea to have a physician okay you for exercise. Also, if you don't have a doctor who takes the time to listen to you, who helps you troubleshoot things that aren't right, and who understands that there is a connection between what you eat and your health, now is the perfect time to find one.

All you have to do to get started with *One Simple Change* is commit to changing one thing. See how it goes, then change another. Remember that it's your body and you are in charge; also remember that nothing in this book is do or die. If you fail at something today, you can still succeed tomorrow. Every time you get up in the morning, you have a new day in front of you, and each new day is a new opportunity for change.

So cheers to change! I sincerely hope this book inspires a positive transformation in your life and in the lives of many others.

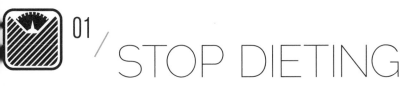

01 / STOP DIETING

IN THE INTRODUCTION, I told you about my miserable experience with dieting. Sadly, I don't think my story is all that unusual; I know many people who have similarly messed up their bodies by restricting their food intake in some way. I also see many people out there who just can't seem to figure out how to eat normally *and* feel comfortable about their weight, so they're always on one diet or another. They are always searching for the diet to end all diets, but they never do seem to find it.

Most diets fail, but even those that seem to work at first do not help you maintain your weight loss (and certainly not your health) over the long term. It's not good for you, nor is it sustainable, to skip meals or drastically cut calories. According to Julia Ross, author of *The Diet Cure* (1999), you need to eat at least 2,500 calories per day to be healthy.

But all calories are not created equal, and I'd really prefer it if you stopped counting calories altogether. Please stop fretting about fat grams, too: Chances are you're not eating enough healthy fat! And while cutting back on carbohydrates can indeed be beneficial for weight loss and health, a diet that eschews them completely isn't recommended (I explain why, and help you figure out which types of carbohydrates to eat, later in the book).

You may not even remember what it feels like to eat without dieting. If that's true, it's time to remind yourself! I don't believe that dieting is healthy for your body or your mind—and I am sure you could use your precious time and energy in much more fun and productive ways. Instead of always worrying about what you think you're not supposed to be eating, I want you to shift your focus to eating without any agenda other than supporting your health.

Please don't ever take healthy eating to an extreme. There's a name for that and it's orthorexia; it can be just as damaging to your body and mind as any sickness. Food should be enjoyed, and meals should be shared with family and friends. If your so-called healthy diet prevents you from doing this, it's not a good diet.

Weight that will not budge despite good nutrition and regular exercise may indicate underlying food sensitivities (more on these in chapter 11), poor thyroid function, adrenal exhaustion due to chronic stress, insulin resistance, or another physiological problem. You can consult a natural health practitioner to help you figure out if you might be dealing with one or more of these issues, but keep in mind that skinny does not necessarily equal healthy. There is far too much emphasis on thinness in our culture, which is particularly damaging to women.

We are all individuals with different metabolic needs. You may have a lactose intolerance, celiac disease, or an allergy to eggs. You may be a lifelong vegetarian or you may really love eating paleo. Please know that I respect you and your choices 100 percent, and if you've found what works for you, then I think that's fantastic. If you have not found what works for you, though, might I suggest letting go of preconceived notions that you must find and follow a certain diet? It's really best to find a lifestyle—not a method of deprivation—that supports your health.

If weight loss is on your wish list, then I'd like you to put your scale away and pull it out only once or twice a month to see how things are going. When you do, I really don't want you to be attached to what you see. Know that when you embark on a new lifestyle such as the one described in this book, you may put on a few pounds at first. This is especially true if you've been on a very low calorie diet for a long time. As your metabolism adjusts to your new way of eating, however, the weight should come off. Trust that it will.

In the meantime, get away from letting a morning weigh-in dictate your mood or what you plan to eat that day. Your weight is not a measure of your health in any meaningful way. I ditched my scale a long time ago, and it was one of the best things I ever did for myself.

There is absolutely nothing wrong with waking up and deciding you're going to eat light because you overdid things the day before, but don't do it just because the scale says you gained a pound. Always remember that your body needs and deserves to be nourished. Go by how your clothes fit and how you feel, not by what the scale says.

» Say good-bye to dieting for good. Most diets don't work, and dieting isn't healthy for your body or your mind.

» Eating too little food isn't going to help you permanently lose weight. Carbohydrates, proteins, and fats are all required by the body, so don't follow an eating strategy that completely eliminates any one of these three.

» Ditch your scale so you can focus on your health, not your weight.

02 / EAT REAL FOOD

YOU ALREADY KNOW THAT I DON'T BELIEVE IN DIETS. I also don't believe there's a single way of eating that's going to work for everyone. We're all different—from our biochemical makeups to our unique cultural backgrounds to our taste preferences.

That said, I do believe that an individualized diet consisting of real food is what we're all meant to put into our bodies. So what's "real food"? Think about what our ancestors ate long ago, when sustenance could only be procured by hunting, fishing, and gathering. Though it's infinitely easier for us to get meals on the table these days, we would all do well to eat similarly natural, unprocessed food.

Real foods include fruits and vegetables (preferably in season, organic, and locally grown, prepared in all different ways); minimally processed dairy products (organic and raw, if possible); fish that's wild (not farmed, and free of mercury or other chemicals); land-animal foods, including eggs (ideally free-range and pastured only); legumes, nuts, and seeds (preferably organic); and fats that are traditional and unprocessed (from both plants and animals). What about whole grains? These can be problematic for many individuals, so I consider them an optional part of a real food diet. I'll discuss all aspects of a real-food lifestyle in greater depth in the chapters that follow.

Real food is what your body has evolved to eat; your body recognizes it and knows how to digest it. It contains the nutrients you need (unlike processed foods, which are nutrient-poor). Real food makes your taste buds sing and satisfies you on a deep level (whereas processed foods foster cravings, food addictions, and emotional eating).

Real food does not come from a box. It does not contain artificial or refined ingredients, added sweeteners, excessive sodium, processed fats, GMOs, pesticides, or other potentially toxic chemical additives. Real food does not come from a fast-food restaurant (or most chain restaurants), either. Real food doesn't contain man-made preservatives; it will spoil unless you take steps to preserve it naturally.

If you're already making an effort to shop the perimeter of the grocery store, purchase food from farmers' markets or farms themselves, and cook the majority of what you eat, then you are probably eating lots of real food. Good for you! If, however, you eat a "Standard American Diet," composed of many processed foods and meals picked up from the drive-through, or even if you eat lots of packaged foods from the health food store, then you're not eating enough real food, and you have some work to do.

Unfortunately, eating food that is not real is all too easy. It's everywhere, it's inexpensive, and if it's what you are used to, then you probably think it tastes good. But a diet of food that's not real is very likely to mess with your body. *Switching to a diet of real food is essential if you want to live long and feel good while you are doing so.*

Do you want to know what I ate today? For breakfast, I had eggs from my backyard chickens scrambled with leftover roasted root vegetables. Lunch was an Asian-style wild salmon and kale soup made with homemade stock from my Thanksgiving turkey, and a big helping of Spicy Lacto-Fermented Pickles (page 100). Dinner was a salad of greens (purchased at a local farm this morning) dressed with olive oil and lemon juice, followed by sliced aged grass-fed beef (from the same farm) sautéed with lots of onions and peppers, and accompanied by a bowl of steamed broccoli tossed with organic butter and sea salt. Dessert was a couple of squares of dark chocolate.

I am concerned about the prevalence of GMOs (genetically modified organisms) in our food supply. Designed to resist insects and diseases, as well as herbicides, GM crops are currently very controversial for health and environmental reasons, and consumers are beginning to demand mandatory labeling of foods that contain them. The "Big Four" GM crops are corn, soybeans, canola, and cottonseed, which are ubiquitous in processed foods. If you want to avoid genetically modified food, do not eat anything that comes in a box, and choose organic whenever possible (organic foods don't contain genetically modified ingredients). For more information on GMOs and how to avoid them, download the Non-GMO Shopping Guide from Mercola. com (http://gmo.mercola.com/ sites/gmo/shopping-guide.aspx).

I give very few recommendations for dietary supplements in One Simple Change *because if you are not dieting and you are eating real food, supplements are rarely necessary. In fact, supplements can do more harm than good. If you have a health challenge, though, certain supplements may be helpful. Consult a licensed naturopathic doctor (ND) or a holistic medical doctor (MD) to help you decide if they are right for you.*

Now doesn't that sound a lot more appealing than diet food or fast food? Real foods are incredibly satisfying, so I don't eat when I am not hungry.

Do you have to spend an exorbitant amount of time in the kitchen cooking in order to eat real food? No, not at all. I'll tell you some of my real-food shortcuts and share some of my favorite (easy!) real-food recipes with you later in the book. Eating real food does not have to be time-consuming; I can honestly say that no matter how busy I am, I can still eat healthy, tasty, real food at just about every meal. Know that I do like to eat out sometimes, and I do grab a slice of pizza with my kids every now and then; if we eat real food approximately 85 percent of the time, then the occasional "non-real food" splurge is just fine.

QUICK REVIEW

→ Packaged and processed foods are linked to just about every health issue that plagues those of us living in the modern world.

→ You need to eat a widely varied diet of fresh, whole, real foods to be healthy. If your diet is less than optimal, make the switch to real foods.

→ Cook real food at home the majority of the time, then don't worry about the occasional non-real food splurge: Aim for 85 percent real food and 15 percent everything else.

03 / DRINK WATER FIRST THING

DO YOU STUMBLE INTO THE KITCHEN IN SEARCH OF COFFEE right after you get out of bed? Or maybe you're a tea person, like me? I am not suggesting you give up drinking caffeinated beverages (at least not right now); I just want you to drink a tall glass of water within ten minutes of waking up—every single day.

Why drink water first thing in the morning? Our bodies are more than 60 percent water and, unfortunately, this makes us quite prone to dehydration. I am actually pretty parched whenever I wake up, but you can be dehydrated even if you don't feel thirsty. Having a glass of water first thing and then drinking more throughout the day will help you avoid health issues that may be related to dehydration. Eating foods that contain water (like raw fruits and vegetables) and drinking additional healthy liquids will help as well. I'll talk in more depth about what you should and should not be drinking elsewhere in the book, but water should always be your first priority.

If drinking water first thing in the morning sounds unappealing, consider that having just one glass of water is associated with a boost in your metabolic rate. The benefits of drinking water in the morning go beyond the physical, though: I find that having a glass of water right after I wake up makes me feel as if I've kicked off the day on the right foot. Since I've done something good for myself first thing, I am more likely to continue to make healthy choices as the day goes on.

The water you drink (and cook, brush your teeth, and shower with) in the morning and throughout the day should be as pure as possible. If you don't have a well, tap water can contain chlorine as well as a variety of contaminants, so you may want to consider investing in a water filter. Filters vary greatly in terms of what they are able to remove; the National Resources Defense

Council has an excellent consumer's guide online (www.nrdc.org/water/drinking/gfilters.asp). If you do purchase a water filter, make sure to change the filter regularly, or it won't do you much good. Also, if you feel strongly about having a filter on your kitchen sink, consider putting one on your showerhead, as well. Your skin is your body's largest organ and, unfortunately, readily absorbs toxins.

I bring a bisphenol A (BPA)–free reusable plastic water bottle with me whenever I leave the house, and I fill it up as needed. (BPA is considered an endocrine disruptor, a chemical that can interfere with the balance of hormones in the body and cause damaging health effects.) This is much more environmentally sound than purchasing bottles of water, since precious oil is used to make plastic bottles. Though they are recyclable, millions of tons of plastic bottles are thrown away every year, and they will never decompose. What's more, there is evidence that much of the bottled water on the market is no more than tap water in disguise (and a 2008 study by the Environmental Working Group concluded that bottled water often contains a wide range of pollutants).

Another reason to have water first thing—even before you have breakfast—is that you may be better off keeping some of your water intake separate from your meals. Many alternative health practitioners advise against gulping large amounts of water with food, because this may dilute your stomach acid or weaken your digestive enzymes. If you feel like you don't digest your foods well, then try backing off on mealtime liquids. Practitioners of Chinese medicine discourage their patients from drinking very cold water for a similar reason (they believe it squelches the "digestive fire").

If you don't like to drink plain water, then try squeezing some lemon or lime juice into your morning water. I find it easier to drink water that way, and water with citrus has a reputation for being an excellent cleanser. Drinking lemon water with a bit of honey first thing in the morning is an old-time home remedy for weight loss. (An alternative is to drink lemony "spa water"—water in which you've also floated berries or cucumber slices and herbs.)

I just don't really buy the old adage that *everyone* needs to have eight 8-oz/240-ml glasses of water every day. We all have different needs for water intake. I suggest consuming lots of fruits, vegetables, and healthy drinks, and listening to your body. Drink water when you are thirsty, and pay special attention to drinking more when exercising vigorously or spending time outside in heat. It's also a good idea to keep an eye on your urine. When you are properly hydrated, it should be very light yellow (though certain vitamin supplements and vegetables like beets do color your urine, rendering it an unreliable indicator).

And what about sparkling water: bad or good? I love the stuff, to be honest, but I only drink it in moderation because carbonated beverages are acidic and can weaken your teeth and bones when consumed in excess. I will discuss this issue further in chapter 34.

Keep in mind that you can, indeed, drink too much water, and that doing so may be dangerous. When you drink far more water than your body needs over a short period of time, you can dilute the concentration of sodium in your blood. Sodium acts as an electrolyte, carefully controlling the fluid balance in our cells. If excess fluid enters our brain cells due to the presence of too little sodium, seizures, coma, and eventually death can result.

The 2003 to 2004 National Health and Nutrition Examination Survey, conducted by the Centers for Disease Control and Prevention, found detectable levels of BPA in more than 90 percent of Americans over age six. It is used in food and drink packaging, including many plastic water bottles and the lids of most food cans. You can limit your exposure to BPA by choosing alternatives to plastic for food and drink storage (I use glass whenever possible) and by not heating food in plastic containers in the microwave. It's also best to limit your use of canned foods, unless the cans are labeled "BPA-free."

QUICK REVIEW

⇨ Drink a tall glass of room-temperature water within ten minutes of waking up. Add the juice of half a lemon or lime for better flavor and potential cleansing benefits.

⇨ Everything you eat and drink affects your hydration: A diet high in fruits, vegetables, and healthy drinks will keep you properly hydrated.

⇨ Sip water throughout the day but don't obsess about drinking eight glasses of water. Listen to your body and drink water when you are thirsty. Keep an eye on your urine (if it's very light yellow, that's good).

04 / GET A GOOD NIGHT'S SLEEP

IF YOU ALWAYS HAVE TROUBLE FALLING ASLEEP, or if you habitually wake up in the night and can't get back to sleep, then you're not getting a good night's sleep. You're not getting one if you toss and turn throughout the night, either. If you've been missing out on some winks, I want you to start getting a good night's sleep.

Deep rest for a good many hours *each and every night* allows us to be at our best every day. When we don't sleep well, things like our concentration, memory, motivation, and mental performance suffer. We also (obviously!) feel tired when we don't sleep well.

Sleep is needed for much more than your mind and energy level, though. It's a time when your muscles and other bodily tissues, as well as your organs, are undergoing restoration. Sleep is also a time when hormones that regulate the immune system, appetite, and rate of metabolism are being produced. I can't get into all the hormones involved (there are too many!), but suffice it to say that not getting enough sleep can actually make you sick. (Poor sleep has been linked to heart disease, diabetes, and depression, for example.) Not sleeping enough can also negatively affect your weight.

For most people, a good night's sleep is the ability to fall asleep right away and sleep deeply for at least eight hours. Some individuals may be able to get away with an average of seven hours per night, but less than that probably isn't enough. If you have a history of sleep deprivation, or a lot of stress in your life, or you are dealing with an acute or chronic health issue, you probably want to strive for an even longer sleeping stretch on a regular basis; you may need as much as ten hours per night. Note that these numbers are what I am suggesting for adults. Children have different sleeping requirements and need to sleep even more.

TIPS FOR GETTING A GOOD NIGHT'S SLEEP

Keep to a schedule. Try to get to bed at the same time and wake up at the same time every day. Establishing a routine makes it more likely that your body will fall asleep easily each night. This is true for children as well, so if your teenager does not have good sleep habits, don't let him or her sleep in too much on the weekend. (I know firsthand that this is very tough to enforce, but it's important.)

Exercise daily. Physical activity promotes good rest at night. If you have trouble getting to sleep, it's probably best to do your workouts some time in the morning so that you're not too hyped up in the evening. I'll talk more about exercise in chapter 6.

Get some sun. Exposure to the sun, preferably early in the day, helps to regulate levels of the hormone cortisol (a high cortisol level in the evening is associated with poor sleep). It also helps with production of the sleep-regulating hormone melatonin. If you live in an area where the sun is not reliable year-round, a full-spectrum light source may be helpful. I'll discuss the benefits of sunlight further in chapter 7.

Sleep in complete darkness. Most of your melatonin is secreted overnight by your pineal gland, but this happens only in complete darkness. For this reason, make sure to keep your room as dark as possible. Heavy shades will help, and so will unplugging or covering up anything that's emitting light in your bedroom, including smartphones and digital clocks. If you do wake in the middle of the night (to pee, for example), it's best not to turn on the light because if you do, your melatonin secretion will stop (not easy, I know—take it slow so you don't bump into anything). It's also best to keep the lights in your home low in the evening, so your body knows it's time to start winding down.

Keep your blood sugar steady. Some people wake in the middle of the night because their blood sugar drops, so follow a blood-sugar-balancing diet, which includes some protein, carbohydrates, and healthy fats at each meal and snack. (I'll talk much more about all of these in later chapters.) You should also limit caffeine in the afternoon, and don't eat a big meal or have a lot to drink right before bedtime. Some people sleep best when they have a light snack at bedtime that contains protein—try it and see if this works for you.

Create a comfortable sleeping environment. Make sure your pillow and bed feel good to you, and replace them if they don't. Seriously—invest in a better mattress if yours is too firm or too soft, or if it's very old. Your bedding can affect the way you sleep, as well; it should be soft, and made from natural materials. Research shows that for optimal sleep, the best temperature for your bedroom is around 60°F/16°C (a bit on the chilly side). Try opening your bedroom windows to let some fresh air in at night, if possible.

Go to bed by 10:00 PM. Some people will sleep better simply by adjusting their sleep routine so they are getting to bed by 10:00 PM and waking up around 6:00 AM. We evolved to go to bed after sundown, so our bodies don't function well when we stay up for hours into the night. If you sleep eight hours beginning at 11:00 PM or later and you still don't feel rested, try going to sleep at 10:00 PM. If you can't get to sleep at 10:00 PM because you're not tired, make yourself wake up at 6:00 AM for a few days no matter what time you went to bed. Chances are you will soon start to feel sleepy at 10:00 PM.

Respect your bed. Don't watch television, use your laptop or phone, or eat in bed; do these activities somewhere else. Reading in bed helps some people relax, but not others (you know who you are!). The only thing you should do in your bed is sleep (and have sex). If you happen to wake up in the middle of the night and have a hard time getting back to sleep, leave the bed for a while to attempt to wind down, and return to your bed only when you're ready to give falling asleep another go.

Take time to wind down. Don't work or do another activity that is likely to stimulate or upset you right before bed; do something that calms your mind instead. Take a tepid bath (the best temperature because it relaxes the central nervous system, according to traditional naturopathic wisdom), read a book, or listen to relaxing music. If you are stressed about something, try putting your thoughts on paper so they're no longer swimming around inside your head.

Nap early. Some people love naps and function better when they take them. If this is you, avoid napping late in the day—finishing your nap by 3:00 PM is best.

Avoid excessive alcohol and pharmaceutical sleep aids. These are habit-forming and have many potential side effects. Some herbs can be very helpful, though; organic lavender oil is a natural sleep aid, for example. Try dabbing a bit on your temples or put a drop on your pillow.

If you cannot resolve your sleep problems on your own, you may have one or more health issues that are keeping you from getting a good night's sleep. Hormonal fluctuations during menopause can cause insomnia, as can many medications. A physician (preferably one versed in natural medicine) can help you sort these things out so you can get the rest you need. He or she will also be able to recommend the right dose of herbs or other supplements—like the hormone melatonin—that may help.

QUICK REVIEW

→ Sleep deprivation is associated with a number of health problems, including weight gain.

→ It's best to get to sleep by 10:00 PM and sleep at least eight hours.

→ If the tips outlined in this chapter do not work for you, consult a health professional so you can get your sleep back on the right track.

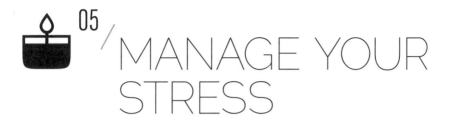

MANAGE YOUR STRESS

ARE YOU ABLE TO ROLL WITH THE PUNCHES, or do the stressors in your life constantly trouble you? Life can be stressful; there is no doubt about that. Stress can come from just about anywhere (for example, your morning commute, your work, your finances, and maybe even your family). The way you manage stress determines how it affects you.

If you have been through or are currently in the middle of a very long and drawn-out stressful situation that is affecting your health, the tips that follow can definitely help. I do, however, also suggest that you seek the help of a health practitioner who can give you an individualized treatment plan for managing your stress.

TIPS FOR MANAGING STRESS

Make sure to get enough sleep. As I discussed in chapter 4, good sleep is essential to good health, and most people do not sleep enough. Sleep is more restorative to the body than just about anything else, and it's a must for properly managing stress. Not sleeping enough is a physical stress in and of itself, and sleep deprivation makes it less likely that you'll be able to handle all that life throws at you. Get at least eight hours of sleep, and more if you are very stressed. Make it a point to go to bed by 10:00 PM (recall that your adrenal glands—the tiny organs responsible for the housing and release of your stress hormones—do their resting between the hours of 11:00 PM and 1:00 AM).

Exercise on a regular basis. Getting the right kind of exercise on a regular basis decreases stress hormones and increases endorphins—chemicals that make you feel good (I try to work out five days a week, and this is why). Note that if you are chronically stressed, however, you should not do very intense exercise because it may adversely affect your stress hormones. Gentle forms of exercise—like slow walking or swimming, and some forms of yoga (not "hot yoga")—are best if you've been very stressed for a long time (more on this in chapter 6).

Pay attention to your diet. When we are stressed, it's common to make poor food choices. I'm sure we've all told ourselves that we "deserve" a pint of ice cream (or a plate of french fries, or whatever) when life has gotten hard— hello emotional eating! Junk food isn't going to alleviate your stress, however; eating lots of it (or falling into other destructive habits, like smoking or drinking excessive amounts of alcohol) is actually one of the worst things you can do for yourself when you're under stress. Stress is rough on the body, so do yourself a favor and support your body with a nutrient-dense real-food diet.

Be careful about caffeine. Even though stress can leave you feeling depleted, guzzling coffee or other caffeinated beverages, such as soda, is not the solution. Your adrenal glands are already taking a beating when you're stressed (they're on overdrive secreting the hormones adrenaline and cortisol). Caffeine only serves to stimulate them further. If you exhaust your adrenal glands, you can end up very fatigued and sick (which will only stress you further), and it will be difficult to recover.

Get to know your limits. Learn how to say "no," so you can keep your life as simple as possible. A less busy life is a less stressful life! Lofty goals can be a source of stress—better to keep your goals realistic and attainable. Don't compare yourself to others and don't try to be perfect; focus on being the best you that you can be.

Breathe deeply. Your blood needs to maintain a pH of 7.35 to 7.45 for optimal function of your cells. When we are stressed, we tend to breathe shallowly at an accelerated rate (we hyperventilate), which makes our blood pH greater than 7.45 (overly acidic). If you focus on taking deep and slow breaths in and out, you can calm yourself down and return your blood pH to normal; give this a try whenever you feel overwhelmed. I often rely on this technique to chill myself out; it can be done anytime and anywhere. Focus all

Is finding time to relax on your own a challenge? If so, I want to encourage you to start scheduling some solo downtime into your days—time when you can just think, and check in with yourself to make sure your needs are being met. I love taking walks alone; I also enjoy cooking alone. I think everyone needs to find his or her own way to spend time alone, even if it's just for a few minutes every day.

your attention on your breathing while you are doing this; if your heart rate is elevated due to stress, taking ten deep breaths can slow it down like magic.

Make time for downtime. Being too busy or working too much really adds to your stress load. Find the time to do relaxing things that you enjoy as often as possible, like chatting on the phone with a dear friend, taking a bath, reading a book, or cuddling with your partner, kids, or pets. I sometimes relax by cooking an elaborate meal for no apparent reason (or by going out for one). And though I don't get to take them as often as I'd like, I am a big fan of vacations in sunny places.

Focus on being mindful or in the moment. This forces you to stop thinking about all the things that are stressing you out, so you can focus solely on what you are presently doing. I talk much more about what this means (and how to do it) in chapter 38.

QUICK REVIEW

⇒ Learn how to effectively manage your stress.

⇒ Make sure to get enough sleep, exercise regularly, support your body with good nutrition, watch the caffeine, and know your limits.

⇒ Deep breathing, scheduling downtime, and being mindful will also help you combat "the stress monster."

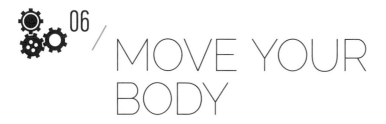

06 / MOVE YOUR BODY

I AM BETTING YOU ALREADY KNOW that exercise is vital to heart health and good overall muscle tone, boosts your mood and immunity, and reduces your risk of cancer and other disease. And as I mentioned previously, exercise is also associated with better sleep and a decrease in your overall stress level. I think we're all aware that exercise is good for us, but did you know that a cardio workout isn't the be-all and end-all?

For a long time, we were told that doing lots of cardiovascular (a.k.a. aerobic) exercise was the key to being healthy, so that's what I did back in my dieting days and for many years after (though I didn't enjoy it at all). I always felt like my body looked the same no matter how much I ran or how many aerobic classes I took, but I still sweated away miserably for the good of my health.

Well, I have changed the way I exercise since I learned that strength training has some pretty remarkable benefits (including an increase in muscle and a decrease in fat; enhanced cardiovascular health; a reduction in muscle and joint pain; increased bone density; and improvement in physical performance, cognitive abilities, and self-esteem). I walk and hike because I enjoy spending time outside, and I occasionally go for a run when I feel like it. I have a black belt in karate, and I ski with my family as often as possible in the winter. But what has really made me more fit (and makes me feel great!) is doing high-intensity conditioning and strength-training workouts. So I focus on these. For a couple of years I did this type of workout with a friend who is a terrific personal trainer. These days, I go to a local CrossFit gym most weekday mornings right after my kids leave for school. It's a different workout every day and I love it.

I firmly believe that for you to get the most out of exercise, you have to find something that you truly enjoy and will want to keep doing. So experiment;

Exercise has many benefits, but exercise alone probably won't help you drop pounds/kilograms. According to Gary Taubes, author of Why We Get Fat *(2010), exercise increases the appetite and as a result, most people end up eating more to compensate for the calories they burn off through exercise. If you revamp the way you eat by following the suggestions in this book and you exercise, however, you may lose weight.*

Research shows that our bodies are genetically programmed to do short bursts of high-intensity exercise (the kind of exercise our ancestors got). But as I mentioned in chapter 5, if you are chronically stressed, you should not do very intense exercise. If you do, exercise can work against you; it can make you fatigued, depress your immune system, and possibly even cause you to gain body fat because of the way exercise affects your stress hormones. So if you are feeling wiped out from stress, you're better off focusing on less intense forms of exercise that are calming and relaxing.

change it up and figure out what you like. Try out a new gym; work out with machines or take group classes to see if you have fun and get something out of them.

Take up hiking if you like to spend time outdoors; biking is another wonderful way to exercise and enjoy nature. Swimming is nonimpact and is excellent for beginner exercisers. And there are many different types of dance classes out there, as well as a variety of martial arts to choose from. Some people are crazy for tennis, others for snowboarding, and still others gravitate toward yoga or pilates. Maybe you'll find you enjoy lots of different things that appeal to you; feel free to do them all! (But I do highly recommend you put some strength training into your exercise program somewhere; you should also stretch your whole body a few times a week.)

If you are currently not an exerciser, then how about just taking a walk every day? Don't think of it as exercise; just think of it as a way to clear your head and get some fresh air and sunshine (if the sun happens to be out). Or you can just think of it as a way to get somewhere. If you constantly profess that you don't have time to exercise, I'm going to call you out on that; just about everyone has time to do something, even if it's just going for a ten-minute walk. The only things you need to go for a walk are some comfortable clothes and good footwear. A buddy (or a dog) to go with is nice, but not required. A friend recently shared that she listens to audiobooks on her smartphone when she's walking, which I think is a great idea.

If it's raining and you can't get outside, then how about taking the stairs instead of the elevator? Or why not put on some music and dance around the house for a while? *If you truly can't find any time in any of your days to exercise, then you need to look at how you can alter your schedule so that's no longer the case.*

→ Move your body almost every day.

→ If you're an avid exerciser but mostly a cardio fiend, consider cutting back and incorporating some strength training into your exercise routine.

→ Make sure you don't overdo the exercise; overtraining can cause real harm, as can doing very intense exercise when you are under chronic stress.

→ Exercise has many benefits, but weight loss isn't necessarily one of them; research shows that the way you eat has a much greater impact on your weight.

07 / GET A LITTLE SUNSHINE

ARE YOU AFRAID OF THE SUN? Do you fear wrinkles and skin cancer so much that you won't spend any time outside without sunscreen? If so, it's not surprising; for a long time, the prevailing opinion among dermatologists (broadcasted by the media) has been that the sun is truly terrible for you.

While it is true that sunburns put you at risk for skin cancer (the ones acquired in childhood are particularly problematic), we're throwing the baby out with the bathwater if we avoid the sun altogether. A little sunshine on our skin can actually do us a lot of good.

Sunshine makes us happy, presumably because sunlight increases levels of the brain chemical serotonin; anyone who's experienced seasonal affective disorder probably understands this connection all too well. The sun positively affects levels of the hormone melatonin, as well. Melatonin combats insomnia, so a little sun can lead to better sleep.

But perhaps most important, exposure to sunlight is directly connected to our vitamin D levels; our bodies make vitamin D when the sun's ultraviolet B (UVB) rays hit our skin. Low levels of this vitamin—which acts a lot like a fat-soluble hormone—are associated with heart disease, certain cancers, strokes, infectious diseases, diabetes (both types), dementia, depression, skin disorders, and a host of autoimmune diseases. Because vitamin D aids in the absorption of minerals, a deficiency can also lead to osteoporosis (calcium cannot be absorbed when there's inadequate vitamin D).

Depending on your skin tone and where you live, approximately fifteen minutes of sun exposure on 25 percent of your body two to three times per week will allow you to meet your vitamin D needs. That's it—not so much. The catch is that UVB rays are only available during midday hours, when the sun is highest in the sky—exactly the time of day we've always been told to avoid the sun. You can't get UVB rays when you're wearing sunscreen, or through a window or smog, and you get little through a cloud cover. Very fair-skinned individuals (yes, redheads, I am talking to you) will require less exposure (probably more like ten minutes). Those with darker skin will need to spend more time outside to reap the sun's benefits (the pigment melanin acts as a natural UVB blocker).

Vitamin D deficiency is extremely widespread these days, yet most people who have it don't even know. The only way to be sure you're getting enough vitamin D is by way of a blood test; ask your doctor to order the 25(OH)D (also called 25-hydroxy vitamin D).

If you've previously avoided the sun, make sure to start with just a few minutes at a time so you can build up some tolerance, but continue to put sunscreen on your face, because it's a small area and the skin is thin and prone to sun damage. Your arms and legs (if you're wearing shorts) can and should be sunscreen-free for the amount of time that you discover is right for your body each day, though. After that, feel free to put on sunscreen if you're going to stay outside for a while.

Please know that I am not at all recommending that you sunbathe for long periods of time each day—that's not good for your skin's health or appearance in the long run. I am also not advocating that you use tanning beds if you can't get out in the sun; as far as I know, they're pretty terrible for you.

You never want to burn, so if you're traveling to a place where the sun is stronger than at home and where you may be outside more than usual, be very careful; you may only need five minutes to get the amount of UVBs you were getting at home. Make sure to use a sunscreen with a high SPF if you're doing the beach thing (though I recently learned that there is no point in going above SPF 50), and make sure to cover yourself or seek shade before you've overdone it.

Remember that it's the bad sunburns (and your genes, unfortunately) that put you at risk for skin cancer; but know that the skin cancers associated with the sun are not usually life threatening. I've actually seen no compelling evidence that deadly melanomas are caused by sun exposure; in fact, it's been postulated that the synthetic chemicals in most sunscreens may be contributing to skin cancers.

Washing your skin with soap right after sun exposure can interfere with vitamin D production, so try to wait a few hours before you do so. Something else you should know: A diet high in antioxidants may offer natural protection against sunburn, so be sure to eat brightly colored fruits and vegetables, dark chocolate, and green tea. Foods high in omega-3 fatty acids (I'll talk more about these in chapter 20) may also be useful in this regard.

If you live thirty-seven degrees north—as I do—you have a problem. (I suggest checking out the chart at www.health.harvard.edu/newsweek/ images/latitude-vitaminD.jpg to determine your location.) There's just not enough sun during the fall and winter for you or me to meet our vitamin D requirements. Upping your intake of foods rich in vitamin D is definitely suggested in this case; unfortunately, vitamin D occurs naturally in only a small selection of foods: free-range egg yolks, raw milk, wild salmon, sardines, mackerel, and organ meats like liver are sources of vitamin D. These foods are not exactly common fare these days, so you may need to take supplemental vitamin D if your levels are low and you don't get enough from the sun and your food.

Another option is to take cod liver oil as a whole food alternative to supplements (I take it every day in the fall and the winter). *Note that you can't overdose on vitamin D from the sun or from food, but you can get too much from supplemental forms (including cod liver oil). It's best to take supplemental vitamin D only under the supervision of your physician.*

QUICK REVIEW

⇢ Sunlight can brighten your mood, help you sleep better, and boost your level of vitamin D; aim to get some sun every day.

⇢ It's best to spend about fifteen minutes in the midday sun; be careful if you are very fair-skinned, so you don't burn.

⇢ If you are low in vitamin D, be sure to include foods that are naturally high in vitamin D in your diet (and consider taking a daily supplement of vitamin D or cod liver oil under the guidance of your physician).

08 / LET IT GO

WHEN MY MIND AND PERSONAL SPACES GET CLUTTERED, I am much more likely to feel anxious and unhappy; it also becomes hard to get things done. Is the same true for you? Clutter can take many forms; I want you to think about what clutter means to you, and how you can start to let it go.

Let's begin with mental clutter. Do you tend to stew over things in your mind? Do you spend time and energy pondering situations you can't change? Do you anguish over certain people's actions, wishing you had some control over them? Do you harbor resentment over past hurts? If so, it's definitely time to work on letting stuff go.

I used to have a real problem with this. If someone did something that made me upset, I'd replay the event over and over in my head. I'd obsess over why this happened. I'd fixate on what I could have done to make things different. I'd be angry, and I couldn't seem to forgive and forget until a significant amount of time had passed.

One day I realized that not letting things go was keeping me stuck in a place of hurt and disappointment. It was also wasting my brain space and time, and it was keeping me from getting important things done. I decided to start letting things go, and I've been a much happier person ever since.

If you don't have any emotional baggage to dump right now (lucky you!), then how about focusing on the physical ways in which you can let some things go? Take a look around your home. Open your closets and your drawers. Are you holding onto things you don't need? Now is a great time to let them go. I promise you will feel so much better when you do. Don't worry about your kitchen and pantry right now, though—we'll get to those in the very near future.

There are entire websites and books devoted to clutter control, and you can even hire a professional consultant to come to your home, so

I am not saying that if something traumatic has happened, you should simply dismiss it and get on with your life. Quite the contrary; I encourage you to do whatever you need to do to process the event. Counseling can be very helpful. But then I encourage you to forgive, since that's the healthiest way to move forward.

You know what else I want you to let go of? Being perfect. The pursuit of perfection isn't worth your time or effort—being perfect is impossible. So let go of trying to have a perfect job, perfect house, perfect family, or overall perfect life, because it's never going to happen. Instead, focus on being the very best you that you can be.

clearly many people must struggle with clutter. I'm definitely no expert, but I've gotten better at clutter control in the last few years by doing two things:

1. **I carefully consider all purchases and don't buy anything unless I really need it (most of the time, anyway!).**

2. **I do not let a week go by without addressing any clutter that's accumulated.**

When I notice that an area of my home needs streamlining or organizing, I attack it right away and work on it until it's done. I get rid of (or move into storage in the basement) anything I haven't used in the last six months. I donate items or sell them on eBay whenever possible, as I hate to throw stuff away. But some things do have to go in the garbage. When that is the case, I avoid thinking about what something cost or whether I might need it someday in the future. These thoughts generally lead me to keep stuff that I shouldn't, and that defeats the whole purpose of uncluttering. I know that labeled storage containers are my friend, but I only keep things in them that truly have sentimental value, or that I am certain I will need at some point.

Another thing I am really conscious of is my e-mail in-box. It's not easy to keep it clutter free, but I find I am much less anxious when I respond to important e-mails as soon as they come in, file things I truly need to save into well-labeled folders, and delete everything else.

QUICK REVIEW

⇨ Learn how to let mental clutter go.

⇨ Let go of trying to be perfect: It's never going to happen!

⇨ Work on the physical clutter in your home, as well. Pare down your possessions so your life is easier to manage.

⇨ Letting go helps to decrease stress.

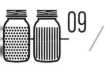

09 / REVAMP YOUR PANTRY

IN THE LAST CHAPTER, I TALKED ABOUT LETTING GO OF CLUTTER. Did you do so? Doesn't it feel good to get rid of all that unnecessary junk? And did you let go of trying to be perfect, too? How does that feel for you?

Now I'd like you to work on your pantry. Since you are on the real-food bandwagon, I encourage you to clear your shelves of everything that isn't real food. Start by taking stock of what you've got. Clear a surface and empty all your cabinets out. Toss everything that's past its prime, along with all the items you know you shouldn't be eating. All packaged and processed foods should definitely go. I hate telling you to throw things away, so if something is compostable (or suitable for donation), please go that route.

A lot of people don't cook much, and consequently don't eat very well, because they just don't keep the right staples in their kitchen. They also eat junk food for snacks, because that's what they have in the house. If this is going on with you, now's the time to make a change. I want you to restock your kitchen with everything you need to create wholesome, nourishing meals for you and those you love.

My goal, when I stock my pantry, is to know that I can throw together a tasty meal with what I have on hand pretty much anytime. I want to be able to make any dish that pops into my head, or that I see online or in a cookbook or magazine, with a very minimal amount of shopping for additional ingredients (like fresh fruit or vegetables, dairy, or meat). The more items I have on hand, the better off I am. So I keep a lot of staples in my pantry.

I've got many different oils and vinegars; dried legumes, like black beans and chickpeas; different types of lentils; grains and pastas; various nuts, seeds, and dried fruits; a variety of unrefined sweeteners and sea salts; and a giant collection of herbs and spices. I've also got a pretty big collection of regular and gluten-free flours for baking. I buy as many of my pantry items as possible in bulk (to save money and avoid packaging), and I store everything that is suitable in glass jars with tight-fitting lids. This works very well for keeping my ingredients organized and away from pests; it also means I can keep as much of my food away from plastic (and its potentially unsafe chemicals) as possible.

I also have a lot of home-canned fruits and vegetables, which I spend time preserving each summer. I make many jars of sauce with tomatoes from my garden, for example. Though homemade jams can end up being pretty high in sugar, I make them with local fruit and derive great pleasure from having them around. I use them in small amounts throughout the winter, and I also give them as holiday gifts.

What about you? Do you have a lot of stocking up to do? Feel free to take your time with this—getting your pantry where you want it to be probably won't happen in one day.

QUICK REVIEW

↪ A well-stocked pantry is the secret to adventurous, delicious cooking. Clean all the junk out of your pantry and restock it so you can make wholesome meals and snacks.

↪ Take time to figure out what you need to have on hand— then go shopping!

↪ Buy in bulk whenever possible, and then store your ingredients in well-sealed glass jars.

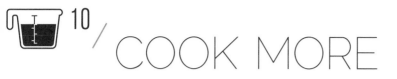

10 / COOK MORE

I LOVE TO COOK. This isn't surprising, since I spent so much of my childhood hanging out (and also working) in my family's restaurant. These days I am both the designated chef of my household and a food writer, so I am in the kitchen more than ever; I really could not be happier.

But I don't want you to think I spend a lot of time making food that is very involved; I don't. I prefer food that is uncomplicated—delicious, but simple—when I eat at home, and so does my family. Ironic as this may seem (considering that I have a recipe blog), I don't even cook from recipes most of the time. I prefer experimenting and being creative in the kitchen. I may not be able to sing or dance or draw, but I can cook.

I see cooking much more as art (and magic) than as science, and I really believe it should be fun. If more people saw it that way—instead of as a chore—they'd be inclined to do it much more often.

Obviously, I think everything in this book is worth doing if you want to be healthier, but cooking real food for yourself and your family should be at the very top of your priority list. If you don't know how to cook, then take the time to learn. Cooking for yourself (or living with someone who cooks) is the very best way to guarantee that you're eating real food.

Food made at home from scratch is much better for you. People who eat out frequently are more likely to consume fewer fruits and vegetables and more unhealthy fats and sugar (and they are likely to weigh more) than those who do not. Moreover, making food at home is cost-effective, and when you cook with real-food ingredients, you're being eco-friendly because you're avoiding excess packaging.

I am a particularly big fan of making a lot of my own staples. It's pretty amazing how many of the things you previously thought you had to buy

You don't need a lot of equipment to cook healthy, tasty, real food. Sharp knives and a couple of cutting boards are important. If I had to choose my favorite pan, it would be my well-seasoned cast-iron skillet. I also use my stainless-steel small and large lidded pots, as well as my giant stockpot, quite a bit. And my wok is well loved, too. Heavy-duty baking sheets are excellent for baking and for roasting vegetables. I don't recommend using cookware with nonstick surfaces made from chemicals like Teflon. They scratch easily, and then potentially toxic particles can get into your food. Worrisome gases can also be released into the air when nonstick surfaces are overheated.

can in fact be made at home. (The irony, of course, is that these foods were always made at home until it became more convenient to buy them.) Two homemade staples that I am never without are chicken stock (facing page) and plain yogurt (page 39); they're so easy to make, you may never buy them again.

What are other foods you can make instead of buy? If you eat bread, consider learning how to bake your own; it's not hard to do (and kneading is a great workout for your arms). Though I don't eat a lot of grains, I do make bread every now and then. I also love transforming local fruit into jams, and I've dabbled in cheese making. I've made my own sausage and cured my own bacon (so I could use organic, pastured pork and avoid potentially carcinogenic nitrites). Heck, I have even made my own Oreos (a.k.a. fauxreos), which are a lot more work than opening a chemical-filled package of my early childhood favorite, but are absolutely delicious.

For many more ideas for things you can make instead of buy, I strongly suggest you pick up *The Homemade Pantry* (2012) by my friend Alana Chernila. It's full of fantastic recipes for easily crafting your own healthful alternatives to packaged staple foods.

QUICK REVIEW

⇥ Eat as much home-cooked food as possible; this is far healthier than eating food made elsewhere.

⇥ If you don't know how to do so already, learn how to prepare your own meals with real-food ingredients.

⇥ Take the time to make your own staples, too. When you make your own food from scratch, it will taste better and it will benefit your health, and you'll save money. It's also more eco-friendly—a win all around.

HOMEMADE CHICKEN STOCK

Makes about 4 qt/3.8 L

When you've got homemade stock on hand, you can make a terrific soup in no time. Chicken stock is also useful for making delectable sauces, and I sometimes sip it on its own as a nourishing beverage. Because it is made from bones, it contains natural gelatin (which is great for the digestive system) and lots of minerals. Adding an acid to chicken stock, like the apple cider vinegar in this recipe, helps draw calcium out of the bones and into the stock.

This recipe is my go-to chicken stock, the one I make when I've got two or three chicken carcasses stashed away in the freezer (left over from roasting chickens or making chicken soup). Feel free to add additional vegetable scraps; sometimes I throw in chopped broccoli stalks, green onion tops, and the like, which would otherwise have ended up in the compost. I do not add salt to my stocks; I prefer to add it to my soups after they've finished cooking.

NOTE: *In this recipe and all the others in this book, please use organic ingredients whenever possible.*

2 or 3 free-range chicken carcasses

1 large onion, *peeled and quartered*

2 or 3 large carrots, *peeled if not organic and roughly chopped*

3 stalks celery with leafy tops, *roughly chopped*

1 tbsp black peppercorns

2 tbsp apple cider vinegar

...continued

1 Combine the chicken carcasses, onion, carrots, celery, peppercorns, and vinegar in a large stockpot, and add water to cover (4 to 5 qt/3.8 to 4.7 L). Bring to a boil and skim off the foam that rises to the top.

2 Reduce the heat and simmer, uncovered, for at least 2 hours or as long as 8 hours, periodically skimming off the foam if necessary. The longer you simmer the stock, the more flavorful it will be. Add hot water as needed to keep the contents of the pot submerged in liquid. When the stock has finished cooking, allow it to cool (you can speed the process by placing the pot in a sink full of ice water). Strain through a colander set over a large bowl, discarding the solids. If you want to skim the fat off (I do not), refrigerate the stock and the fat will congeal at the top, making it easy to remove.

3 Your stock is now ready for use. Or you can pour it into containers and put them in the freezer. (I store mine in 1-qt/960-ml BPA-free plastic containers; glass jars can also be used for freezer storage and are a healthier option, but please use caution in stacking them so they don't crack.) Chicken stock will keep for 1 to 3 months in the freezer.

TURKEY STOCK

Increase the amounts of everything in proportion to the larger size of the turkey carcass. (You'll end up with many quarts/litres of stock, so make sure you have enough room to store them.)

VEGETABLE STOCK

Load up your pot with any vegetables that you have on hand, omit the chicken and vinegar, and add enough water to just cover all the vegetables. Simmer the stock for 45 minutes to 1 hour.

HOMEMADE YOGURT

Makes 1 qt / 960 ml

Yogurt made with live cultures is high in protein, calcium, and probiotics, which aid the digestive system. I'm a big fan of low-tech yogurt making; you don't need any fancy equipment to make wholesome plain yogurt.

Herbalist Susun Weed recommends consuming 1 qt/960 ml of organic yogurt each week to strengthen the immune system and prevent cancer. I eat my yogurt plain or with nuts and dried fruit or a few spoonfuls of homemade granola. And I also add it to smoothies.

You can use any kind of milk, but for the most healthful yogurt, use the most healthful milk you can find. I suggest organic, preferably raw cow's milk, or goat's or sheep's milk. Full-fat milk will make the richest, thickest yogurt; the fat in yogurt helps your body assimilate the calcium and other nutrients it contains.

4 cups/960 ml milk

1 tbsp plain, live-culture yogurt

EQUIPMENT

One 1-qt/960-ml glass canning jar with a screw-top lid, *metal or BPA-free plastic*

...continued

1 Clean the glass jar and lid in hot, soapy water, or use the hottest setting on your dishwasher.

2 In a small pot, heat the milk over medium heat to a temperature of 180°F/82°C. If you don't have a kitchen thermometer, heat the milk until it is just starting to boil; don't let it come to a rolling boil as this will be too hot. Make sure you don't walk away from the milk and allow it to boil over, because it makes a big mess (trust me). Use a slotted spoon to remove any skin that forms on the surface of the hot milk.

3 Remove from the heat and let the milk cool to 110°F/45°C, about 25 minutes. (You should be able to put a fingertip in the milk and hold it there for 10 seconds.) Put the pot into a bowlful of ice water to speed the cooling, if you'd like. Don't let the milk cool below 110°F/45°C; it needs to be at this temperature to culture properly.

4 Pour the milk into the canning jar and gently mix in the yogurt. Cap the jar tightly. Preheat your oven to 110°F/45°C. Once it reaches this temperature, turn it off. If you can't set your oven to 110°F/45°C, preheat it to the lowest setting possible (in many ovens, this is 200°F/95°C), and then turn it off and give it time to cool down until approximately 110°F/45°C.

5 Wrap your jar in a thick towel (I use a big bath towel) and place it in the oven on its side (remove racks as necessary so that it fits). Turn the light of your oven on (to keep it warm) and close the door.

6 The towel will insulate the jar, ensuring that the milk stays warm during the culturing process. Leave it there for about 12 hours (or at least overnight). Unwrap the jar and place it in the refrigerator to cool for several hours. You now have homemade yogurt!

7 If you end up with liquid (the whey) floating atop your yogurt, mix it in or, for thicker yogurt, pour it off. Don't discard the whey, though; it contains water-soluble vitamins and minerals, as well as protein, and can be added to soups or used in other recipes. Homemade live-culture yogurt will keep for 1 to 2 weeks in the refrigerator; you can use 1 tbsp of your homemade yogurt to make another batch.

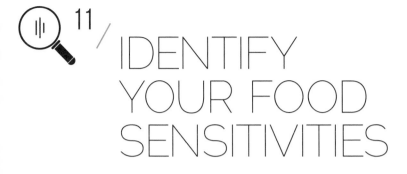

IDENTIFY YOUR FOOD SENSITIVITIES

IF YOUR DIET HAS BEEN LESS THAN OPTIMAL, or you eat the same foods all the time (or both), then you may have food sensitivities. You may even be eating something that does not work for your body if you've been consuming a good diet of real foods for a while. It is important to become aware of any food sensitivities you may have if you want to optimize your health.

What are food sensitivities? Sometime they're referred to as food allergies, but I don't like to use that term. Most people associate food allergies with an immediate immune system response—the kind of situation that causes you to break out in hives or that results in anaphylaxis (think life-threatening peanut allergy) right after you eat a food. Food intolerances are a bit different from food sensitivities, as well; these generally stem from an enzyme deficiency (as is the case of lactose intolerance) or possibly from a weakness in the digestive system. Celiac disease has some characteristics of an allergy because the immune system is involved, but it's generally defined as a complete gluten intolerance.

Food sensitivities appear to involve the immune system, but they don't usually cause reactions that are immediate. And you are not born with the propensity to develop food sensitivities, as is the case with food allergies and intolerances. Food sensitivities generally develop because you eat certain foods too often or because your digestive system or immune system isn't as strong as it could be. A diet too low in healthful fats can also predispose you to food sensitivities.

Food sensitivities cause inflammation throughout the body and can negatively affect your health in numerous ways. They may cause abdominal bloating from an accumulation of gas and can also often lead to fluid retention, which makes you look puffy.

Food sensitivities can cause many other symptoms: fatigue that does not resolve despite good quality sleep, respiratory issues, skin disorders like acne, recurrent infections, excessive mucus production, joint pains, headaches, PMS (premenstrual stress) and other hormonal problems, dark circles under the eyes, and mood disorders such as anxiety or depression are all possible indications of food sensitivities. If you are dealing with one or more of these symptoms, they may be clues that you are eating foods to which you are sensitive.

Now I know what you must be thinking: If you are not getting an immediate, strong response from your body after you eat a food (the kind that happens when you have a true food allergy), then what's the harm? And aren't there many other possible reasons to explain why you could have the symptoms listed above?

The fact that your symptoms may be hard to connect with the foods you are eating does not mean you should ignore them. And just because many women you know have PMS does not mean it's an unreliable indicator of food sensitivities. Food sensitivities are really quite common; once you remove the offending foods from your diet, you may be amazed at how much better you feel.

When I was in college, I became sensitive to wheat, dairy, and sugar because those were the foods that I ate all the time (they also happen to be the most common offenders when it comes to food sensitivities). When I stopped eating them, I was able to lose weight in a very short period of time because the water I'd been retaining for years simply disappeared. Lots of people don't believe me when I tell them that I lost 15 lb/6.8 kg in three weeks (I am a petite person, so it would seem impossible). But if you understand that it was a "deflation" that was going on, and not fat loss, then it does make sense.

So how do you know if you have food sensitivities, and what do you do about them? Interestingly enough, you are likely to crave the foods that you are reacting to; this is because food sensitivities cause a situation not unlike drug or alcohol addiction. Does the thought of going without bread for even one day send you into panic mode? If so, then you may be sensitive to wheat. If you can't bear the thought of not being able to have ice cream every night after dinner, that's an indication that you may be sensitive to dairy. Consider that what you perceive to be an issue of willpower may be more akin to a true physiological addiction—one that you can stop once you aren't eating the foods to which you are sensitive anymore.

In addition to wheat, dairy, and sugar, other commonly reactive foods include eggs, soybeans, peanuts, corn, tomatoes, and strawberries. Food additives and dyes can also cause reactions in some people. I know it's hard to believe, but you could even be sensitive to something like carrots if you happen to eat them all the time.

If you think you may have a food sensitivity, take the food that you suspect *completely* out of your diet for two weeks. (Some health practitioners say you only need to remove the food for four days, but two weeks is better because it ensures all traces of the food are out of your system.) If you have no idea what food may be to blame, look at one (or more) of the foods you consume most often. When it's no longer in your system, do you notice a difference in how you feel? After two weeks, eat some of the food *by itself* and *on an empty stomach* and pay close attention to any reactions. Did symptoms that had begun to resolve themselves come back? Did you get a bellyache or a blast of congestion or fatigue? It can be helpful to take your pulse before and after you eat the food; if your pulse quickens after you eat it, then you are most definitely sensitive to that food. This process of identifying food sensitivities by eliminating foods from, and later reintroducing them into, your diet is called an elimination and challenge.

If there's a possibility that you have multiple food sensitivities, you may be better off getting a blood test for food sensitivities, rather than playing around with eliminating and challenging foods on your own. A holistic medical provider will be the best person to help with this, since many traditional medical doctors still do not acknowledge that food sensitivities even exist. I find this last point confounding, to say the least, given my experience. Considering how often we put food into our bodies, doesn't it make perfect sense that sometimes foods can cause problems? Something that's healthy for someone else may not be healthy for you.

If you do turn out to be sensitive to a food, it does not necessarily mean you can never eat it again; your body might just need a break from it. If the problem isn't too severe, you may get over your food sensitivity after a relatively short period of complete elimination (try six to twelve months). Or you might be able to tolerate eating small amounts of the food, but only on occasion. On the other hand, you might need to avoid the problematic

Many detox diets—including juice fasts—lead to an increased sense of well-being not just because they promote the release of toxins from your body but also because you are not eating foods to which you may be sensitive while you are following the diet. I have done these in the past, but nowadays I am more interested in creating a healthy lifestyle for the long haul than in forcing myself to detox for any length of time. If you think you might benefit from a brief, healthy detox diet, though, I recommend the book Clean *(2009) by Alejandro Junger.*

food for a good long while and work with a holistically inclined doctor to strengthen your immune system. (A diet of real foods high in antioxidants and healthy fats—particularly the omega-3 fatty acids—can be very helpful.) Supporting your digestive system will also be key (I talk more about healthy digestion in chapter 27). Once you heal your food sensitivities, it's important to eat a varied diet and rotate your foods, so you don't end up with the same problem again.

QUICK REVIEW

⇨ Food sensitivities are different than typical food allergies and food intolerances.

⇨ Sensitivities are remarkably common, and any food can be a culprit (wheat, dairy, and sugar are the top offenders).

⇨ If you have symptoms that you have not been able to resolve, try an elimination and challenge diet on your own, or speak to your natural health care provider about food sensitivity blood testing.

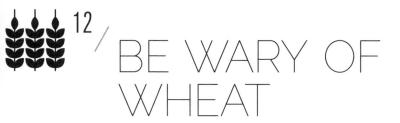

12 / BE WARY OF WHEAT

MANY PEOPLE (ESPECIALLY IN THE UNITED STATES) eat wheat at just about every meal and in every snack. This isn't hard to do if you have cereal for breakfast, a sandwich for lunch, pasta or pizza, additional bread at dinner, and crackers, cookies, or other wheat-based treats in between—wheat is everywhere! Even if you make a concerted effort to eat a healthy, somewhat diversified diet, you probably still eat some wheat.

We've been led to believe that as long as we're avoiding wheat in its refined form most of the time, there's nothing wrong with eating lots of it, but I beg to differ. As I mentioned in the previous chapter, wheat is one of the top offenders when it comes to food sensitivities, but that's not the only reason I think you should be wary of it.

The wheat in our food supply has changed drastically since humans first started practicing agriculture. Over time, wheat has been manipulated in countless ways in efforts to create a high-yield, disease-resistant grain. The end result is a product that's much lower in protein and much higher in gluten and a number of other problematic components than our ancestral wheat. Because modern wheat is consumed in great amounts by such a great many people, it's really no surprise that it appears to contribute to a great many health problems. According to William Davis, the author of the book *Wheat Belly* (2011), modern wheat consumption is linked to obesity, diabetes, joint problems, osteoporosis, skin disorders (including acne), and heart disease. Wheat is also the main source of gluten in the human diet, so if you have celiac disease, it can make you very ill (more on celiac disease in chapter 13).

After I took wheat out of my diet, long before books like *Wheat Belly* were on the bestseller lists, people would generally eye me suspiciously when

I told them I didn't eat it. Twenty years later, I still eat wheat on a pretty limited basis. (Fortunately, it's much easier these days to avoid wheat because there are so many alternatives on the market, and no one looks at you funny anymore.)

Even after so many years of limiting my wheat consumption, I find that if I eat a small amount, I end up wanting more. This makes sense, since wheat appears to have an addictive component; it also seems to act as an appetite stimulant for me. I know I can get higher quality carbohydrates and far more vitamins and minerals from other foods like fruits and starchy vegetables, so it's a no-brainer for me to eat wheat in small quantities.

If you haven't yet removed wheat from your diet, I want to encourage you to do so now. Even if you were skeptical about the whole food sensitivities discussion, why not try going without wheat for a week or two anyway? What do you have to lose? Sometimes you don't realize how bad you were feeling until you start to feel well. Try going without wheat to see if it makes a difference in your energy level, your weight, or any symptoms you may have; you may be surprised by what happens. (And if you experience no change in your health, at least you'll have explored some new foods.)

If you have no interest in going wheat free (or if you try the elimination and challenge and ultimately decide wheat works just fine for you), then I still suggest cutting back, because wheat has a reputation for exacerbating inflammation in the body. And choose properly prepared health-promoting forms of wheat when you do eat it. True sourdough bread, made by soaking and fermenting wheat (or sometimes rye), is probably the healthiest bread to eat. It is also worth seeking out sprouted-grain tortillas and cereals should you choose to eat these foods, as they are much better for you. You should also look for products made with the ancient form of wheat known as Einkorn, which is much more healthful than regular wheat and is less likely to cause reactions, since it has not been hybridized and contains less gluten.

→ Modern wheat is linked to numerous health issues, including obesity, diabetes, joint problems, osteoporosis, skin disorders (like acne), and heart disease.

→ If you eat a lot of wheat, go wheat free to see if your health improves.

→ If you don't want to go wheat free (or if you try it and find that you were doing just fine with wheat), then consider eating less, and seek out healthier sprouted-wheat products and foods made with Einkorn wheat.

13 / CONSIDER GOING GLUTEN OR GRAIN FREE

AS I DISCUSSED IN THE PREVIOUS CHAPTER, many people feel loads better when they stop eating wheat (or eat less). You may want to go a step further, however, and eliminate (or at least limit) gluten and possibly all grains; let's talk about why.

Gluten is a protein that's found not only in wheat (and its "ancestors" spelt and Kamut) but also in barley, triticale, and rye. It's also found, though to a lesser extent, in oats. Gluten is what gives breads made from wheat their structure, their unmistakable doughy-ness.

When I was growing up, I didn't know anyone with celiac disease. Nowadays, however, I know lots of people who have it. Why the shift? Well, for one thing, it was clearly underdiagnosed for a long time. I've spoken to several friends who had long-standing health issues, realized as adults that they had celiac disease, and went gluten free. They no longer suffer from their old symptoms. Also, as I mentioned in the previous chapter, the wheat in our diets has changed; there is more gluten in wheat now than ever before.

Celiac disease is an autoimmune disorder characterized by a complete intolerance to gluten. Like many other autoimmune conditions, celiac disease and less severe forms of gluten intolerance can be either genetically or environmentally acquired. Some people develop gluten intolerance because of chronic stress or acute trauma in their lives, while others end up with it due to an already compromised digestive system, possibly as a result of over-medication with antibiotics, which destroy the normal bacteria in the gut. It's also possible that feeding grains to infants before their digestive systems are ready to handle them may set the stage for gluten intolerance down the road.

If you have celiac disease and you eat gluten, your body will treat it as a toxic foreign substance and attack it. This causes inflammation, which damages the lining of your small intestine. Continuing to eat gluten will damage your small intestine even further, until it can no longer absorb nutrients the way it is supposed to. This will weaken your immune system and may cause you to become ill in a variety of ways. Early symptoms of celiac disease usually include bloating, abdominal pain, diarrhea or constipation, and steatorrhea (an abnormal amount of fat in one's stools). But I have a dear friend whose main symptom was migraine headaches. If you have any of these symptoms, talk to your doctor right away.

You should get tested for celiac disease and get a proper diagnosis before you try cutting gluten out of your diet. (If you have celiac and you go gluten free before getting tested, the test will likely not be positive.) Celiac disease is a serious medical concern, and the only cure is strict, lifelong gluten avoidance. If you have celiac disease and you go on a permanent gluten-free diet, your intestines will heal and you will become healthy again.

It is estimated that approximately 1 percent of the population has celiac disease, but that a far greater percentage of people have a gluten sensitivity; this is why it's wise to consider going gluten free even if you don't have celiac disease, or at least consider eating a limited amount of gluten.

People who are sensitive to gluten may have digestive symptoms (like gas, bloating, and constipation). Gluten sensitivity can also cause many nondigestive health problems. As I mentioned in chapter 11, food sensitivities, including a sensitivity to gluten, can cause symptoms like acne, joint pains, depression, and fatigue—the types of symptoms you might deal with for a long time without figuring out the cause. It is likely that only after you stopped eating gluten—and the symptoms went away— would you make the connection. Note that people with gluten sensitivity don't test positive for celiac disease.

Keep in mind that just because you are experiencing a health issue does not mean you are definitely sensitive to gluten. You might be sensitive to wheat but not to all foods with gluten, or you might

It's practically impossible to completely avoid gluten unless you are preparing foods yourself in your own kitchen just about all the time. I recommend cooking at home for everyone, but if you have celiac disease, it's even more important to know how to prepare real food (or to live with someone who does). If you eat any processed foods at all, and if you eat out (except at a dedicated gluten-free establishment), you run a very high risk of ingesting gluten. It's necessary to be vigilant, since eating even the tiniest amount of gluten—a single crumb of bread, for example—can make you very sick. Be aware that gluten lurks in many places you would not expect it; some medications, vitamins, and herbal supplements use gluten as a binding agent, and lipsticks and even postage stamps may contain gluten, as well.

be sensitive to something entirely different in your diet, such as dairy, or soybeans, or anything else that you consume on a regular basis. Or maybe your problem doesn't stem from food sensitivities at all; maybe you don't sleep enough and that is why you're always tired! I am mentioning this because I see a lot of people these days who apparently think going gluten free is a cure-all for everything, including being overweight. This is not necessarily the case; in fact, if you have celiac disease you may gain weight when you go gluten free because your body will finally be able to properly absorb all the nutrients from the foods you are eating. I'm not saying going gluten free isn't valuable for those who have a gluten intolerance or sensitivity—it is! But going gluten free isn't the answer to every single health or weight problem.

If you suspect you have a sensitivity to wheat, but after giving wheat elimination a try you don't end up feeling any better, then consider going gluten free. If that doesn't cut it, then consider going completely grain free.

People following a paleo lifestyle avoid all grains, and many report success not just with weight loss but also with healing metabolic disorders and autoimmune conditions. Though initially I dismissed paleo as just another diet, I don't think attempting to re-create the way our very distant ancestors ate is a bad thing at all—there are a lot of positives that can come from it, actually.

Now, what if you are in very good health with no signs of sensitivity to wheat, gluten, or grains—can you eat as much of these foods as you want? Or what if you tried avoiding wheat, gluten, or grains, but it made absolutely no difference in how you feel—what then?

If you fall into one of the above camps and you don't buy into the paleo theory that all grains are bad for everyone, there's really no reason to practice complete grain avoidance. That said, it's wise for us all to keep an eye on the grains in our diets, because they are high in carbohydrates that elevate insulin levels, and they are often produced with agricultural practices that are contributing to environmental degradation.

If you are going to eat grains, then eat a variety of them, preferably soaked first. Soaking grains makes them easier to digest, and gives our bodies greater access to their nutrients. (Soaking helps to neutralize phytic acid, a naturally occurring compound in grains, legumes, nuts, and seeds that makes it difficult for your body to absorb the minerals contained in these foods.) For the healthiest oatmeal, for example, you should soak your oats overnight in a mildly acidic liquid (such as water mixed with a little yogurt or lemon juice). Discard the soaking water and cook them in fresh water the next day.

Gluten-free grains like rice, and seeds like quinoa and millet, can be cooked without soaking, but Sally Fallon, the author of *Nourishing Traditions*, believes these foods should be soaked, too, in order to neutralize their phytic acid content. Note that if quinoa is soaked for long enough (twelve to twenty-four hours), it starts to sprout and generally becomes soft enough to eat without cooking, so the enzymes are preserved, and it remains a raw, living food. If you do want to cook your seeds and grains, though, make sure to discard the soaking water and cook them in fresh water. Note that they will cook faster after soaking.

One last cautionary note: Be careful about overdoing it with treats. Eating too many sugary carbohydrates—even if they are wheat, gluten, or even grain free—is not healthy for anyone (more on sugar in chapter 14). If you have celiac disease or a gluten sensitivity, gluten-free baked goods won't wreak havoc on your digestion the way gluten-containing foods would. But you'll be far better off if you focus primarily on eating foods that are naturally gluten free (like protein foods, dairy products, fruits, vegetables, legumes, and nuts and seeds).

QUICK REVIEW

→ Know the symptoms of celiac disease and get tested by your doctor if you think you may have it.

→ Some people are sensitive to gluten without having celiac disease; you will feel better avoiding gluten if this is the case for you. And some people might want to eat no grains at all because this will make them feel best.

→ If you try avoiding wheat and other grains but find it makes no difference whatsoever in the way you feel, then go ahead and enjoy these in small amounts. Try foods like oats, rice, quinoa, and millet (soak them first, and then cook in fresh water, in order to digest them well).

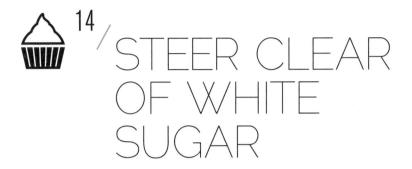

14 / STEER CLEAR OF WHITE SUGAR

BACK IN MY LOW-FAT-EATING DAYS, I craved and ate sugar pretty much constantly as long as it wasn't accompanied by fat. Nonfat frozen yogurt was my very best friend and we hung out every day—sometimes more than once. I had to give up sugar completely (because it was one of my food sensitivities) for about a year, and I've been very careful about consuming it ever since.

How do you know if you are someone who needs to cut back on sugar? Well, if you have extremely strong cravings for it and can't stop eating sweets once you start, then I'd say you have a sugar problem, wouldn't you? If you know you have insulin resistance, then you definitely have a problem with sugar, as well. But you may have other issues that you do not connect with your sugar consumption, like mood swings, fatigue, and frequent yeast infections.

You probably already sense that sugar is addictive, and I bet you know it's not great for your teeth (the bacteria responsible for cavities feed off sugars). But did you know that sugar may depress your immune system, and that too much sugar in the diet contributes to a host of issues, including acne, digestive problems, food sensitivities (see chapter 11), yeast overgrowth and infections, and even cancer? Also, when your body processes sugar, your own stores of vitamins, minerals, and enzymes can be depleted.

Sugar is a very concentrated source of carbohydrates, and eating it raises your insulin levels. Chronically high insulin contributes to weight gain as well as a host of health problems, including heart disease and diabetes. Excess sugar consumption also appears to shrink the brain, cause depression, and very possibly lead to Alzheimer's disease.

Processed foods and packaged drinks are very high in sugar (often in the form of high-fructose corn syrup). One 12-oz/360-ml soda contains more than 3 tbsp. You may be getting much more sugar than you realize, even if you buy packaged foods that are marketed as healthy. Manufacturers add sugar to replace the fat in low-fat foods; many brands of granola and yogurt have quite a bit of added sugar, too. Read the labels! If you are eating real food—and I hope you are—then you don't need to worry about this (see chapter 2 for a review). Know that it's easy to make these foods yourself if you are so inclined; I have a bunch of different refined sugar–free granola recipes on my blog. And do check out the Homemade Yogurt recipe on page 39.

Fortunately, there are many sweet pleasures out there that do not contain any sugar at all. There are fresh and dried fruits, of course, plus there are a number of vegetables that are naturally sweet: Winter squashes, carrots, beets, and other root vegetables all come to mind. These are real foods that contain vitamins, minerals, and fiber; they satisfy the desire for something sweet without damaging your health.

What should you use when baking or otherwise sweetening foods at home? I suggest exploring the range of natural (and preferably organic and fair-trade) sweeteners on the market, such as whole cane sugar, coconut sugar, raw unprocessed honey (this is one of the reasons why I have my own bees), real maple syrup, and molasses. I also use traditional sweeteners like jaggery and palm sugar on occasion, as well as organic fruit juice. All of these are less refined or processed than white sugar (they also contain some minerals so they are not completely empty calories). I used to like agave, but then I started reading bad things about how processed it is and about how much it raises your blood sugar, so I don't use it anymore. If you still feel okay about it, make sure to look for organic raw agave.

High-fructose corn syrup (HFCS) is really bad news, and should always be avoided. Derived from cornstarch, HFCS is added to many processed foods because it's very cheap (large corn producers receive government subsidies). There is evidence that our bodies handle fructose even more poorly than the sucrose in white sugar (made from cane or beets). Moreover, most corn grown in the United States is genetically engineered.

There are many other unrefined sweeteners that I haven't mentioned here; if you want to try them out, make sure to choose ones that have undergone minimal processing and do not go overboard with them. It's really best to limit all desserts to a couple of small servings a week, especially if weight loss is one of your goals.

Know that your body can still react negatively to natural sweeteners if you have a sensitivity to sugar. You might want to give one of the sugar-free, low-carbohydrate sweeteners (such as stevia) or one of the sugar alcohols (such as erythritol or xylitol) a try. I don't like the way stevia tastes and I have no experience with the others, but I have heard good things from diabetic friends who use them (but note that the sugar alcohols can potentially cause digestive discomfort).

Artificial sweeteners are not a good substitute for sugar because these are about as far as you can get from a real food. They may have no calories, but they don't seem to decrease the desire to eat sugar (for some people, they actually exacerbate sweet cravings), and they don't seem to help with weight loss, either. Also, despite their prevalence in our food supply, I honestly don't trust that they are safe. I'll talk more about artificial sweeteners in the context of quitting soda in chapter 34.

QUICK REVIEW

⇒ Cut back on the sugar you consume, particularly white sugar.

⇒ Eat naturally sweet foods—such as fruit and root vegetables—instead of sugar.

⇒ Explore the range of unprocessed sweeteners on the market and bake your own desserts with them—then eat in moderation.

15 / FIND YOUR CARB BALANCE

MANY PEOPLE EAT WAY MORE CARBOHYDRATES than they actually need. A diet that's too high in carbohydrates (especially refined and sugary ones)—and consequently low in protein and healthy fats—will raise your blood sugar and insulin levels. This can lead to a spectrum of health problems, ranging from relatively benign (for example, vague malaise) to very serious (cardiovascular disease and diabetes).

You will likely benefit from decreasing the total amount of carbohydrates you consume while simultaneously increasing protein and healthy fats. Bringing your diet into balance in this way can help you reverse issues related to high insulin. It can also help you lose weight (if you have weight to lose) and improve your health overall.

Cutting back on the carbohydrates you eat can also make a difference if you deal with fluctuations in your energy level and sugar cravings throughout the day; these are both indications that your blood sugar levels are all over the place. Most people reach for carbohydrate-rich comfort foods when they're feeling fatigued, but this just makes the problem worse. (Eating regularly throughout the day also helps a lot; I talk more about that in chapter 17.)

While I do suggest you dial the carbohydrates back—and you may have already done so by eating less gluten, wheat, and other grains—as I mentioned in chapter 1, I do not think you should eliminate carbohydrates completely. Though low-carb diets do help some people lose weight and feel healthier than they did when they were eating a highly processed, high-carbohydrate diet, I want you to get away from dieting, remember? Also, the highly respected endocrinologist Diana Schwarzbein (author of numerous books, including *The Schwarzbein Principle*, 2004), cautions against eating too few carbohydrates, because this negatively affects the chemicals in your brain and your hormones, and can damage your overall health. The more active you are, the more carbohydrates your body will require.

So what kind of carbohydrates should you be eating? Well, we've already focused on how wheat and other grains are really an issue for a great many people. Though they are often suggested as a healthy source of carbohydrates, and whole grains do contain fiber and B vitamins, I don't think they should make up a large part of your diet, even if you don't have sensitivities or intolerances to gluten, wheat, or other grains. At the very least, I suggest minimizing foods made with white flour (including pasta), because they're not very nutritious, they're very high in carbohydrates, and they're made with problematic wheat (see chapter 12). If and when you do eat carbohydrate-rich foods like noodles, try to choose those made with Einkorn wheat or a wheat alternative, and be sure to eat them with protein and healthy fat, so they don't raise your blood sugar too much.

Carbohydrates that don't provoke a big spike in blood sugar are excellent. Many vegetables fit the bill here and are a great choice because they are high in vitamins and minerals; they're also a good source of fiber. Some of my favorites are asparagus, broccoli, cabbage, cauliflower, celery, cucumber, all greens (more on these in chapter 26), eggplant, green beans, mushrooms, peppers, and summer squashes. Beets, carrots, parsnips, turnips, red potatoes, sweet potatoes, and winter squashes are extremely tasty; these are higher in carbohydrates but are still very healthy.

Fruits are a good source of high quality carbohydrates, as well. They're an excellent way to satisfy a sweet tooth and include apples, apricots, avocados (yup, they're a fruit), bananas, berries (all kinds), cherries, figs, grapefruits, kiwis, lemons, limes, mangoes, melons (all kinds), nectarines, oranges, papayas, peaches, pears, persimmons, pineapples, plums, pomegranates, and tomatoes (yup again, a fruit, not a vegetable). Just keep in mind that a few fruits (such as bananas) are much higher in carbohydrates than the others, and for some people, eating too many without enough protein and fat can lead to blood sugar issues.

→ Experiment until you find your own personal balance of protein, carbohydrate, and healthy fat consumption within the larger realm of a real-food diet; you may feel better if you eat fewer carbohydrates.

→ Instead of focusing too much on the carbohydrates you're not supposed to be eating, pay more attention to the things you probably don't eat enough, like non-starchy carbohydrates, protein, and healthy fats. Use the other types of carbohydrates (starchy vegetables, and grains if they work for you) to round your meals out and as occasional treats.

→ Make sure not to limit your carbohydrates too much, however, especially if you are very active. If you don't eat enough carbohydrates, your metabolism will be adversely affected.

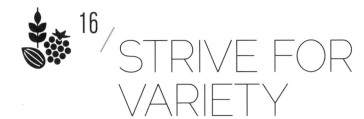

16 / STRIVE FOR VARIETY

DO YOU BUY THE SAME FOODS every time you go to the grocery store? Do you eat the same breakfast every day? How about lunch? Does your dinner plate look strikingly similar each evening?

Eating the same foods each and every day can be problematic, no matter how healthy you believe those foods to be. For one thing, repetitively eating certain foods may cause you to develop sensitivities to those foods (as I discussed in chapter 11). Also, you are more likely to get bored with a real-food diet if you always eat the same things.

The best way to avoid developing food sensitivities and stave off dietary boredom is to eat a wide variety of foods. Alternating different fruits and vegetables, grains, fats, and proteins (both plant- and animal-based) each day (or at least every couple of days) also ensures that you are taking in a wide variety of nutrients.

Am I saying that you should not eat the same thing for lunch that you had for dinner the night before? No, not at all; in fact, I don't want you to stop doing anything that helps you eat well and makes your life easier. I just want to point out that if you are accustomed to eating cereal with milk for breakfast every morning, maybe a turkey sandwich for lunch every day, and an apple for a snack every afternoon, you should consider changing things up.

Why not try to eat as many different colored whole real foods as you can? The more colors you eat, the more nutrients you get. Brightly colored foods, such as berries, are particularly high in antioxidants that protect the cells in our body from damage by free radicals. Free radicals are unstable particles that occur normally in the body, but certain lifestyle habits (like smoking) increase them. Free-radical damage is linked to the development of cancer and other chronic diseases.

I believe that if you eat local foods in the same season in which they are grown, you will naturally eat a more varied diet. Ever since I started gardening, I gorge on tomatoes during the summer months but mostly go without them during the winter (supermarket varieties shipped in from who knows where are a far cry from the ones I grow myself and just aren't worth eating). With each change in season, I explore new fruits and vegetables, such as asparagus in spring and berries in summer. Unless I am noshing on something that I preserved myself—and there's really nothing like busting open a jar of plum jam made in August on a cold day in February—I generally let the season dictate my menu.

QUICK REVIEW

> Eating a varied diet is an excellent way to get the maximum amount of nutrients. It's also a good way to decrease the possibility of developing food sensitivities, stave off dietary boredom, and help support planetary biodiversity.

> Try different grains, herbs, legumes, nuts, seeds, and spices; cook up a dish from a cuisine you don't know much about.

> If you like to bake, experiment with different flours and natural sweeteners.

> If you're vegetarian or vegan, do not rely exclusively on soy for your protein needs. Moderate amounts are fine, but avoid processed soy products, which often masquerade as health foods. (And avoid all soy if you have a thyroid problem or an iodine deficiency.)

Many vegetarians and vegans use foods made from soybeans to meet most or all their protein needs, but overconsumption of soy products may suppress the thyroid gland and cause hormonal disruption in susceptible individuals. If you have any type of thyroid condition, or an iodine deficiency, avoid soy. Otherwise, eat soy in moderation, preferably in traditional, fermented forms (such as tempeh and miso). Avoid processed foods made with soy (including protein powders), as these have an unnaturally high isoflavone content, which can cause health problems. I'd also avoid non-organic soy products because they were probably made from genetically modified soybeans. Vegetarians should eat free-range eggs and organic dairy, plus other protein-rich plant-based foods (such as legumes, nuts, and seeds). If you are vegan, your choices for protein are more limited.

It's becoming clear that industrialized agriculture's practice of relying on just a few crop varieties has contributed to a loss in planetary biodiversity. It is in our best interest to purchase a wide variety of foods. If you garden, choose open-pollinated seeds (those that are pollinated by natural means, such as insects, birds, or the wind) and heirloom seeds whenever possible.

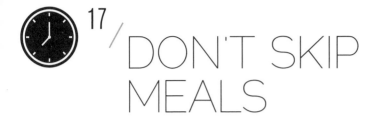

17 / DON'T SKIP MEALS

I ONCE BELIEVED THAT THE LESS I ATE, the better off I'd be. I skipped meals all the time in the interest of keeping my weight down. It was an ill-fated strategy.

Blood sugar balance is vitally important to both weight loss and optimal health. When you diet by restricting your food intake, you lower your blood sugar. When you also skip meals or go for long periods without eating a good snack, you cause your blood sugar to drop even more. If you then eat a large meal that's not balanced (one that's high in carbohydrates, with little protein or fat), it will cause your blood sugar to shoot up rapidly, but then drop down low again. So it's best to eat three meals a day, and to have substantial real-food snacks (which are much like small meals) if you get hungry in between.

Our bodies do best when we eat every few hours. Eating three meals a day (and having snacks when your body needs them) engenders stable blood sugar levels. This means you won't have to deal with issues like shakiness, fatigue, and an inability to think clearly because your blood sugar is getting too low in between meals. It also means you won't be getting so ravenous that when you do eat, you eat too much.

If you've been diagnosed with hypoglycemia (low blood sugar), the best thing you can do is eat very frequently. Some of you might even need to have a little snack every hour or two; if you do this for a while, your blood sugar will stabilize and you can go back to eating less frequently. Make sure these snacks contain protein and fat, and not just carbohydrates. Eating carbohydrates alone (especially refined or sugary ones) in an effort to balance your blood sugar will only worsen the problem.

⇨ Skipping meals will not help you lose weight. It will screw up your blood sugar (making you feel shaky, fatigued, and unable to think clearly). Plus, when you do eat, you'll be more likely to overeat if you skipped the meal before.

⇨ Snack if you get very hungry between meals, but not if it makes you too full to eat at mealtimes.

⇨ Meals (and snacks, if you eat them) should be balanced; they should contain some high quality carbohydrates, proteins, and healthy fats.

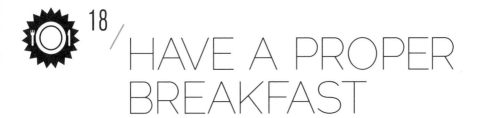

18 / HAVE A PROPER BREAKFAST

DO YOU EAT BREAKFAST? It does seem to be the most commonly skipped meal, so I want to tell you why it's so important to eat it, and what you should have.

You might be surprised to hear this, but until recently, I really struggled with eating breakfast. I'd never wake up hungry (probably because I skipped breakfast for so many years when I was dieting), so it didn't feel good to me to eat anything first thing in the morning. I worried about this because most health experts do feel that breakfast shouldn't be ignored; your blood sugar is very low after fasting overnight, and it's best to eat as soon as possible. Not eating breakfast can also slow your metabolism and set you up for problems with blood sugar regulation.

The thing is, there isn't really any hard evidence that people who eat breakfast are healthier than those who don't. In fact for some people, eating breakfast makes them hungrier throughout the day than if they'd skipped it, which can translate to eating more overall. Another interesting fact: Skipping breakfast every now and then can be considered a form of intermittent fasting (IF).

Studies show that IF helps to boost one's levels of human growth hormone (HGH); increased HGH is associated with a decrease in body fat and may contribute to a deceleration of the aging process. IF appears to work best when you are already in excellent health and when the fasting is followed by high-intensity exercise. Therefore, if you are extremely healthy and eat a high quality real-food diet the rest of the time, it's not going to harm you (and it might even benefit you) to skip breakfast on occasion.

If, however, you are working on getting healthier, have skipped breakfast a lot in the past, have problems with your blood sugar, or are pregnant or breastfeeding, then you should eat a balanced breakfast. It should be composed of some protein, carbohydrates, and healthy fat—a meal that will nourish your body and keep your blood sugar stable until lunch—and you should eat it shortly after you get up. If you really don't like to eat right after waking, then wait about forty-five minutes before you do.

If you don't wake up hungry, try to eat dinner on the early side (no later than 7:00 PM), and avoid nighttime snacking; I'm sure you know that if you eat too much too late at night, you're likely to wake up still feeling full in the morning. You may also need to force yourself to eat breakfast for a while until your body gets used to the habit, and begins to expect food in the morning. I personally fixed my aversion to eating breakfast when I committed to going to my gym in the mornings. For the first two weeks of this routine, I wasn't hungry but still made myself eat breakfast before I went because I did not want to work out on an empty stomach. After two weeks, I started to feel hungry in the mornings, and now I really look forward to breakfast.

You already know not to eat meals that are very high in carbohydrates, and this is particularly true in the morning. It's no shocker that donuts do not qualify as a healthy breakfast, but a bowl of cereal isn't a good choice either. Most breakfast cereals on the market (even the ones advertised as healthy) are made with grains and are pure carbohydrates; they're also highly processed and contain many undesirable ingredients. And anything you pick up at a fast-food drive-through is definitely not a good bet; fast food is low quality and is not real food (and meals eaten in the car are very poorly digested).

So what should you eat for breakfast? Well, I eat something different pretty much every day. Sometimes I'll have gluten-free toast piled high with wild smoked salmon and greens; other days I'll have a small amount of home-made granola sprinkled into a bowl of organic plain yogurt. Or maybe I'll have yogurt with berries, or scrambled eggs on a corn tortilla with chopped avocado and fresh salsa, or a fruit smoothie to which I've added nuts, yogurt, and a raw egg yolk for protein. On weekends, my husband often makes his specialty—breakfast potatoes—which I'll have with eggs and a little bacon (from pastured pigs). See the pattern here? I always make sure to eat some protein balanced with carbohydrates and fat in the morning. Occasionally I will eat a gluten-free scone or another treat that I baked, but I eat just a small amount along with protein and maybe some fruit.

➔ Eat within forty-five minutes of waking up. If you don't wake up hungry and never eat breakfast, force yourself to eat breakfast anyway; after a while, you will wake up hungry and you'll look at breakfast as a pleasure, not a punishment.

➔ Coffee and refined carbohydrates alone are not a balanced breakfast; have a combination of protein and healthy fat along with whatever type of real-food carbohydrates work for you.

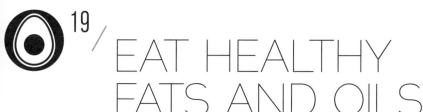

19 / EAT HEALTHY FATS AND OILS

DID YOU KNOW THAT FAT PROVIDES ENERGY AND INSULATION, and that your body uses it to make cell membranes and hormones and to reduce inflammation (which helps with all types of allergies)? And did you know that certain fats, the omega-3s, can also protect you from cancer and keep your heart healthy? Were you aware that fats are necessary for your digestive system to help you absorb certain vitamins, mainly the fat-soluble vitamins A, D, E, and K? Is it news to you that low-fat diets rarely contain enough healthy fats to sustain health, and that people who follow them over a long period of time often end up sick?

I don't think there's any topic under the umbrella of nutrition that's more confusing to people than how much fat to eat, and which fats and oils are healthy and which are not. This chapter is one of the longest in the book because I've a lot to say on this subject.

Up until the early part of the twentieth century, natural fats were the only fats available; they were appreciated for making food taste good, and for their health benefits (fats contain a number of nutrients that are absent from all other foods). In the middle of the twentieth century, however, when shortening and margarine were invented, and cheap vegetable oils—such as those made from soybeans and corn—began making their way into the food supply, the public's perception of fats changed. People started believing these newer processed fats were somehow better for them than natural ones.

In the 1980s, when I was a teenager, everything I read about nutrition said that fats made you fat, and that animal fats were terrible for you. I decided that butter was evil and I would not eat it (or anything made with it). I wouldn't touch anything that contained coconut oil, either; I read that it was a saturated fat and that saturated fats raised cholesterol and caused heart disease. I stayed away from all foods that naturally contained fat and cholesterol, too, such as whole milk, meat, and eggs.

It's unfortunate that at the time of this writing, most people still think they should be eating a diet that is low in fat, particularly saturated fat. I'm not sure why this continues to be the case. Mounting scientific evidence confirms what our ancestors instinctively knew: Many fats (including saturated fats) are actually quite health-promoting.

Now, I can't tell you exactly how much fat you need in your diet. Everyone is different. Due to genetics, some people need more fat than others. If your ancestors lived on the coast (or on an island), you might benefit from eating more because you are descended from folks who ate a fatty fish–based diet.

If, on the other hand, your ancestors were landlocked hunter-gatherers who relied on lean game meats for much of their sustenance, you might need less fat. But either way, I can tell you which are the best fats to eat, and which ones you should avoid.

Medium-chain triglycerides (MCTs) are a special kind of fat, which is easily digested (and therefore helpful for anyone with any kind of digestive disorder) and quickly converted into energy. MCTs can actually boost your metabolic rate. Organic coconut oil is a good source of MCTs.

The best fats to eat are natural fats, including organic butter and coconut oil, whole-fat coconut milk, and the fats in pastured dairy products (including cultured dairy, such as cheese and yogurt), eggs, and grass-fed meat (including bacon from pastured pigs). You can also feel free to eat avocados, pure olive oil, nuts and seeds (and their oils), and the fats you'll find in healthy fish (more on these in chapter 22).

What about for cooking? For sautéing, stir-frying, and roasting (techniques that require heat ranging from low to high, but not as high as for deep-frying), the best choices are fats and oils with a long history of traditional usage. These are fats and oils whose chemical structure allows them to remain stable when heated, such as butter, organic coconut oil, and olive oil.

Use organic grass-fed butter if you can find it, because it's full of vitamins and a special fat-burning nutrient called conjugated linoleic acid (CLA). Butter is also an excellent fat for baking. If you can't get grass-fed butter, or you just can't justify spending the money on organic butter, then it's still better to use regular butter than synthetic butter substitutes and processed vegetable oils.

Once maligned because it's a saturated fat, coconut oil has recently received a lot of positive press for its health-conferring and weight-reducing abilities. I just adore it; I use it in dishes with an Asian flavor profile (such as stir-fries and Asian soups and stews), and I like experimenting with it in baked goods, too. It's also great for cooking eggs. The only drawback is that it does have a somewhat pronounced coconut flavor that not everyone loves (my husband, for example, is not a big fan). That said, if you enjoy the taste but are still wary about using butter or coconut oil, know that these are the best fats to ingest if you have blood sugar issues (even better than olive oil).

Olive oil has always had a reputation for being healthful, even when butter and coconut oil were bashed, but many people don't really understand how to use it. The common perception is that olive oil is not suited to high-heat cooking, but this simply isn't true. Olive oil has long been used for every type of cooking in Spain and other countries. This makes sense because standard pure olive oil (not extra-virgin) has a high smoke point. I personally use olive oil quite often in my kitchen. I cook with it daily and bake with it on occasion.

Note that to preserve the healthful properties of olive oil, it's very important to bring it up to higher temperatures slowly. If the oil starts to smoke, it's too hot and may be harmful to you if consumed because free radicals have been produced. If this happens, you should discard it and start again. Olive oil is not appropriate for deep-frying. (I use the more fragile, and extremely tasty, extra-virgin olive oils for making salad dressings and for drizzling over soups and other cooked dishes.)

Many health enthusiasts who have taken to blending greens into their smoothies may not realize that some of the nutrients in the greens are best absorbed when they are eaten with healthy fats. For this reason, I add some full-fat yogurt, avocado, nuts or nut butters, or maybe some coconut oil whenever I make a green smoothie.

What about grapeseed, peanut, and sesame oils? Until recently I was using grapeseed oil for deep-frying (which I do on rare occasions), but I decided to stop using it altogether because it's rich in vitamin E, which really shouldn't be heated, and because grapeseed oil may be genetically modified. Now, whenever I do deep-fry something, I use lard from pastured pigs (tallow would be another good choice; it is a very stable natural fat). Peanut oil is high in omega-6 fatty acids, and most people already consume too many of these, but it too is fine for occasional cooking and frying. Sesame oil is better drizzled over foods than used as a cooking oil because it's pretty fragile, and what you're really after is its wonderful intense taste, which gets lost when you cook with it.

Flaxseed, almond, and walnut oils are perfect for using cold; these are best in salad dressings and drizzled over cooked dishes. These oils are fragile; they should not be heated, and should be as fresh as possible. Flaxseed oil, in particular, must be kept refrigerated and should be used within a month or so of opening the bottle because it goes rancid quickly. A high quality flax-seed oil will always have the bottling date and the "best before" date printed on the label. As for flaxseeds themselves, I think these are best ground fresh and used raw; using them in the occasional baked good is fine, too.

Macadamia, pumpkin seed, and rice bran oils are fine for cooking at moderate temperatures. Avocado oil is yet another oil that is suitable for cooking (I was surprised to learn that avocado oil has a pretty high smoke point). Make sure that any oils you buy are cold-pressed and unrefined, and aren't made from GM crops.

Despite what you might have read in mainstream nutritional literature, soybean, corn, canola, sunflower, and safflower oils are not very healthy. These oils (and combinations of them, which are labeled as generic "vegetable oil") are highly processed. They have been refined, bleached, and deodorized. What's more, they are unstable and easily damaged by heat, and they appear to lower HDL ("good") cholesterol and contribute to cancer. Also, these oils are typically made from genetically modified crops. If you really want to use one of these oils, buy organic and do not cook with it over high heat.

Keep in mind that these vegetable oils are found in all packaged and pro-cessed foods. Organic vegetable oils are found in many packaged health foods, as well, and while these will at least be GMO-free (which is definitely a good thing), I still think they are best avoided because they're not health-promoting.

You should also make sure to avoid the hydrogenated fats or trans fats found in margarine, partially hydrogenated oils, and fried foods. These industri-ally produced fats are vegetable oils that have been converted into solid fats. They are truly terrible for you because they raise your insulin levels, your LDL ("bad") cholesterol levels, and your blood pressure. Excess consumption of these fats is linked to the development of diabetes, heart disease, and cancer.

QUICK REVIEW

⇥ Eat foods like avocados, egg yolks, full-fat dairy products, whole coconut milk, and fatty fish.

⇥ Use fats such as butter, coconut oil, and olive oil for cooking.

⇥ Avoid refined vegetable oils and unnatural hydrogenated fats. The best way to ensure you are consuming healthy fats and oils is to stock your kitchen with them and do your own cooking.

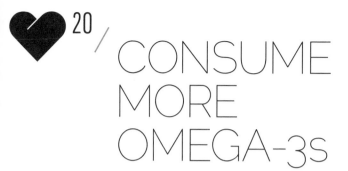

20 / CONSUME MORE OMEGA-3s

IN THE PREVIOUS CHAPTER, you learned why you shouldn't fear natural fats and oils. Now I want to tell you more about one type of fat that we should all focus on getting more of: the omega-3 fatty acids.

A deficiency in omega-3s is connected with everything from type 2 diabetes to heart disease and cancer. Not eating enough omega-3s can also lead to a slow-as-molasses metabolism and depression. Omega-3 fats decrease inflammation in the body, help to balance your hormones, promote proper functioning of the immune system, and foster healthy hair, skin, and nails.

You've probably heard the omega-3 fats (along with the omega-6s) referred to as essential fats. This is because our bodies cannot make them; they must be obtained from food. Unfortunately, omega-3 fats are way harder to get through the diet than the omega-6s.

Omega-6s are found in nuts, seeds, beans, and grains; they're also in the vegetable oils that go into a vast array of processed snack foods (which, as I said in chapter 19, I don't recommend). Commercial eggs, poultry, and meats are all high in omega-6s, too (because commercial animals are fed grains). I think it's easy to see why most people are probably getting way more omega-6s than they need.

Omega-3s, on the other hand, are found in a much smaller, less commonly consumed group of foods. They are plentiful in fatty fish that live in cold water (such as salmon, tuna, mackerel, herring, anchovies, and bluefish). They are also found in sardines (small oily fish related to herring). And you can get omega-3s from the egg yolks of pastured chickens and the beef of grass-fed cows. Sadly, many people are still avoiding all egg yolks and beef because they've been led to believe these are bad for you.

Can you get omega-3s in your diet if you don't eat animal foods? Technically, yes. There are actually three fatty acids in the omega-3 "family." They are alpha-linolenic acid (ALA), eicosapentaenoic acid (EPA), and docosahexaenoic acid (DHA). ALA is found in a variety of foods, and decent amounts can be sourced from plant-based ingredients such as flaxseeds, walnuts, and hemp seeds and their oils; chia seeds; and certain green leafy vegetables, including the "weed" purslane. Unfortunately, on its own ALA appears to be of limited value for your health. (The body is able to convert some of the ALA into EPA and DHA, but this conversion is not very efficient.)

EPA and DHA appear to be much more beneficial; these are the fatty acids that are found in fish such as salmon, pastured eggs, and grass-fed beef.

If you avoid animal foods that contain omega-3s (or if your diet is simply lacking in omega-3 foods), consider taking an omega-3 supplement, so you don't become deficient in this important fat. If you are vegetarian or vegan, you can look into algae oil; otherwise, you can take fish or krill oil.

I don't suggest you run out and buy any old omega-3 supplement from the drugstore or supermarket, though; many of those are neither safe nor effective. (I keep a frequently updated list of the brands that I like on my blog, along with other resources that I recommend, at www.healthygreenkitchen .com/resource-guide). Note that fish oil and fish *liver* oil are not the same thing. Unlike fish oil, fish liver oil—generally made from cod and sometimes from skate—does not generally have high amounts of EPA and DHA, as fish oil does (though fish liver oil is high in vitamin D).

QUICK REVIEW

⇥ Most people eat far too many omega-6 fats, so you probably need to decrease the amount of those that you eat while simultaneously bumping up the omega-3s.

⇥ Eat fatty fish, meat from grass-fed cows, and eggs from pastured chickens, along with dark leafy greens, walnuts, and flax, hemp, and chia seeds.

⇥ If you do not eat many of these foods, consider taking an algae or fish (or krill) oil supplement that's been deemed pure and effective by a reputable third party.

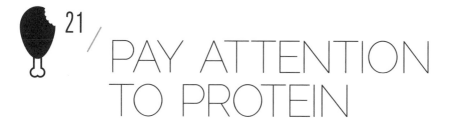

21 / PAY ATTENTION TO PROTEIN

I LEARNED THAT IT'S BEST TO EAT SOME PROTEIN WITH EVERY MEAL and snack when I was in naturopathic school, and I've subscribed to this practice ever since. Protein is really important because it plays a number of structural roles in the body (including the maintenance of muscle mass). It's also essential to the formation of antibodies, enzymes, and hormones, and it helps you balance your blood sugar. Need another reason to pay attention to protein? It keeps your metabolism running strong. Our bodies don't store protein, so we really must eat some every day for protein to be able to do its work.

I want to zero in on the connection between protein and balancing your blood sugar. This is a really key point, and it's the reason why I recommended you have some protein with breakfast every day back in chapter 18 (your blood sugar is particularly unsteady after fasting overnight). If you struggle with sugar cravings—or cravings for any type of carbohydrate, really—then cutting back on carbohydrates (especially those that are refined) and having some protein at breakfast (and then throughout the day) should make a big difference. Having enough healthy fat in your diet will help you balance your blood sugar, as well.

How much protein should you eat for meals and snacks? I personally try to have 15 to 20 g of protein at meals (including breakfast), and about half that amount when I have a snack (though, to be honest, I don't snack that often). I am 5 ft/152 cm tall, and I am pretty active; feel free to adjust these numbers up or down based on your size and activity level. Some may find they need a bit less, and others will need more. If you are eating a lot less protein than this and you're not feeling great, you should definitely try adding more protein to your diet throughout the day and see how you do.

I am not at all suggesting you eat a super high-protein diet; what I am asking you to do is make sure you eat a moderate amount, along with moderate amounts of good quality carbohydrates and healthy fats. To give you an idea of what 20 g of protein looks like: It's the equivalent of about 3 oz/ 85 g of meat, poultry, or fish, 2 oz/55 g of hard cheese, or 3 eggs. A cup of yogurt has about 9 g of protein, and Greek yogurt has twice as much (18 g!). I don't actually weigh or measure anything to make sure I am getting a specific amount; I've been eating this way for so long that building meals around the amount of protein that works for me is just second nature.

I feel best when I am eating some of my protein from animal foods. This could be because I have blood type O; there's evidence that we just don't make good vegetarians (folks with blood type A seem to have a better time avoiding animal foods). But I do eat plant foods that contain protein, such as nuts and seeds, as well. (Most nuts and some seeds contain less protein and more fat than animal foods, so I think they're really best used as occasional snacks and not as your protein source during meals; they're also generally high in omega-6 fatty acids, and, as you'll recall from previous chapters, most people eat too many of these.) Some seeds actually cook up like grains and can be a very nice addition to the diet, whether you're vegetarian or not. Two tbsp of chia seeds contain more than 4 g of protein; ½ cup of cooked quinoa contains approximately the same amount.

Cooked beans and lentils contain between 10 and 20 g of protein per cup; these are very good sources of protein for vegetarians, as are soy foods such as tofu and tempeh. (But recall from chapter 16 that consuming too many soy foods may suppress thyroid function; tempeh appears to be less of a concern in this regard because it is fermented.) Some grains contain a little protein, and so do some vegetables. I don't recommend you eat a lot of those vegetarian packaged foods that are advertised as being high in protein; they are highly processed. I also don't recommend you consume protein powders or protein bars very often; these really aren't whole foods and often contain a lot of questionable ingredients.

→ Protein plays many important roles in the body; it is important to eat enough.

→ Some folks require animal protein to be healthy, while others may do all right without it. Experiment to see what works for you.

→ Choose whole, not processed, sources of protein, and if you eat animal foods, seek out wild fish or pastured animals that were raised humanely. If you are a vegetarian, be cautious about the overconsumption of soy (particularly unfermented soy).

COCONUT TEMPEH AND VEGETABLE STEW

Serves 4

If you are not familiar with tempeh, allow me to make the introduction: Tempeh is a traditional Indonesian soybean product. I prefer tempeh to tofu because it's made from healthier fermented soy, and because it undergoes far less processing. Tempeh is high in protein and fiber, plus it lasts for a while, so I try to keep an unopened package in the refrigerator at all times.

Feel free to swap out the vegetables I've used here for your favorites; pretty much anything works in this stew. I like to top this with some Spicy Lacto-Fermented Pickles (page 100).

---

2 tbsp coconut oil

One 8-oz/225-g package tempeh, *cut into 1-in/2.5-cm cubes*

1 tbsp minced garlic

1 tbsp minced ginger

1 jalapeño or other chile pepper, *minced*

One 13½-oz/400-ml can unsweetened coconut milk *(I like Native Forest brand because the cans are BPA-free)*

1 medium eggplant, *peeled if not organic and cubed*

3 cups broccoli or cauliflower florets (about 8 oz/225 g)

1 cup torn bite-size pieces of kale

2 tbsp brown sugar or coconut sugar

2 limes, *halved, for serving*

2 tbsp minced fresh cilantro *for serving*

All-natural fish sauce (omit for a vegan dish) *for serving (optional)*

Sriracha sauce *for serving (optional)*

1 In a soup pot, warm the coconut oil over medium heat. Add tempeh cubes and cook for 4 to 5 minutes, stirring frequently, until they are evenly browned.

2 Reduce the heat a bit and add the garlic, ginger, and jalapeño. Add a little water to the pot if it looks dry, and cook for about 1 minute more.

3 Add the coconut milk, 1⅔ cups/ 400 ml water (use the empty coconut milk can to measure it), eggplant cubes, broccoli florets, kale, and brown sugar. Stir well and bring to a boil. Reduce the heat and simmer for 25 to 30 minutes, or until the vegetables are very tender.

4 Squeeze a lime half over each portion of stew, sprinkle with a little cilantro, and drizzle with a little fish sauce (I love its unique flavor, but it's not for everyone) and Sriracha (for additional heat), if desired.

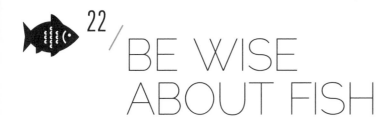

22 / BE WISE ABOUT FISH

FISH HAS BEEN AN IMPORTANT PART OF THE HUMAN DIET for many thousands of years. It's tasty and extremely nutritious, and can be an excellent source of protein, vitamin A, vitamin D, and omega-3 fatty acids.

It's so sad that these days, instead of just happily making a meal out of fish or seafood, we must worry about a host of issues: Has the fish or seafood we'd like to eat been exposed to contaminants, including mercury? Is it a species that's been depleted due to overfishing? Is it farmed or wild, and which is better?

I've considered not eating any fish at all, but since omega-3s are so essential for good health, I don't believe this is the answer. Also, I think it's really important to support local fishermen, as well as those connected to the fishing industry, who are doing the right thing so that fish and seafood are more healthful and sustainable.

The Mercury Problem

Many types of fish and seafood now contain harmful levels of mercury as a direct result of the pollution of waterways from coal-fired power plants. Ingesting high amounts of mercury is very dangerous, as it can damage the brain and nervous system. Unborn babies and young children are particularly susceptible to mercury poisoning.

I always refer to the Natural Resources Defense Council (NRDC) when I want to see where a particular fish stands in relation to environmental contaminants. According to the NRDC, the following types of fish and seafood contain the smallest amount of mercury: anchovies, butterfish, catfish, clams, crab, crawfish (a.k.a. crayfish), croaker (Atlantic), flounder, haddock (Atlantic), hake, herring, mackerel (North Atlantic), mullet, oysters, perch (ocean), plaice, pollock, salmon (canned and fresh), sardines, scallops, shad (American), shrimp, sole (Pacific), squid, tilapia, trout (freshwater), whitefish, and whiting. (However, eating flounder, haddock, scallops, and shrimp is still problematic because their wild populations are low due to overfishing.)

Lobster, cod, snapper, halibut, and tuna are on the NRDC's Moderate Mercury list. The NRDC recommends eating no more than six servings per month of these, and it is probably best if pregnant women and children under the age of four avoid them altogether.

The least healthy fish with the highest mercury count (most of which are also caught using environmentally unsound methods) are king mackerel, marlin, orange roughy, shark, swordfish, tilefish, and ahi (a.k.a. bigeye) tuna. It is best to avoid eating these altogether.

Canned light tuna has less mercury than white albacore tuna; white albacore is on the High Mercury list along with bluefish, grouper, Spanish mackerel, Chilean sea bass, and yellowfin tuna. Fish in this category should not be eaten more than three times per month (children should not eat them more than once or twice per month).

The Overfishing Problem

Some of the low-mercury fish and seafood that would otherwise be recommended for their health benefits are no longer considered sustainable. We should avoid eating these for the most part until their populations have had a chance to recover. As I mentioned above, these are flounder, haddock, shrimp, and scallops. To see the rest of the fish and seafood that are in trouble, please consult the NRDC's online Consumer Guide to Mercury in Fish at www.nrdc.org/health/effects/mercury/guide.asp and take note of the red-starred items. The Blue Ocean Institute's website (blueocean.org/programs/sustainable-sea-food-program/) also has extensive information about sustainable seafood choices.

Wild Versus Farmed Fish

Salmon is my favorite fish. I love the way it tastes, and the fact that it's high in omega-3 fatty acids is a big bonus. Thankfully, salmon is on the NRDC's Least Mercury list.

I only eat wild salmon because farmed salmon are raised in pens, are artificially colored, and may contain toxic levels of industrial chemicals. I no longer buy Atlantic salmon, as it's nearly impossible to find Atlantic salmon that is wild. At this time, the very best wild salmon comes from Alaska. Fish farms have never been allowed there and the water is pristine, so the salmon population is robust. I must say that when I see packaged salmon labeled as wild at the grocery store, I am a bit skeptical; I believe the best place to buy wild Alaskan salmon is from a fishmonger that you trust, or from a company that sells flash-frozen wild Alaskan salmon. I highly recommend the wild salmon and other fish and seafood available at Vital Choice Seafoods and Organics. Visit their website at www.vitalchoice .com/shop/pc/home.asp.

Avoid most other types of farmed fish and seafood (including shrimp and trout), as well; the fish are fed low quality diets, and runoff from fish farms contaminates the marine ecosystem. But there are a few exceptions to the wild-only rule. Commercially available mussels, clams, oysters, and bay scallops are not wild, but the Environmental Defense Fund has deemed them both healthy and eco-friendly. While these do come from farms, they are harvested with suspension nets, which do not harm the ocean or its other inhabitants.

As for tilapia, I've never liked it because I don't think it has any flavor and because it's low in omega-3s. Tilapia farming is a huge business and appears to be harming the environment; I suggest you avoid tilapia, too.

I recommend downloading the Seafood Watch Pocket Guide from the Monterey Bay Aquarium (there is also a free app) to help you decide which fish in your region are the healthiest to eat. You can find it here: www.montereybayaquarium.org/cr/cr_seafoodwatch/download.aspx.

QUICK REVIEW

⇥ For unlimited consumption, choose wild Alaska salmon and sardines.

⇥ For moderate consumption, stick to the fish and seafood that are not high in mercury and have been deemed sustainable.

⇥ The Seafood Watch Pocket Guide from the Monterey Bay Aquarium will help you decide which of the fish available in your region are the best to eat.

SARDINE SALAD

Serves 1 or 2

My family runs for the hills when I open a can of sardines, so I generally eat this salad for lunch when I am home alone. I love how quickly it comes together, how nutritious it is, and how it sustains me for the entire afternoon. Unfortunately, just about every brand of commercial mayonnaise is made with soybean or other undesirable oils, so here are your options: Look for mayonnaise made with olive oil (extremely hard to find), make your own olive oil mayonnaise (easier than you think), or use the highest quality mayonnaise you can find. As for the sardines, I prefer the water-packed ones, but the olive oil–packed ones are also fine; make sure the brand you buy does not use BPA in the lining of the can.

Eat the salad as-is; over salad greens; on an open-faced sandwich made with whole-grain or gluten-free bread; or with whole-grain, gluten-free, or nut- or seed-based crackers (I love it with rice crackers).

One 4⅓-oz/125-g can wild sardines

2 tbsp minced green onion (white part only) or red onion

3 to 4 tablespoons fresh lemon juice

Freshly ground black pepper

1 cup/100 g diced cucumber

½ ripe avocado, *diced*

2 tbsp diced celery

2 tbsp diced red or yellow bell pepper

1 to 2 tsp mayonnaise, *preferably made with olive oil*

1 Mash the sardines in a bowl with the green onion. Add the lemon juice and black pepper to taste, and mix well. Add the cucumber, avocado, celery, bell pepper, and mayonnaise. Mix to combine.

O²³/ EMBRACE EGGS

DO YOU FEAR EGGS? If so, I don't want you to be afraid of them anymore, because they are among the most nutrient-dense foods you can eat. Eggs don't cause heart disease and there's probably no reason for you to limit them in your diet, especially if you enjoy them. The key is to choose eggs of the highest quality in order to take advantage of all the nutritional benefits they offer.

Cholesterol was identified as a cause of heart disease back in the late 1950s by a researcher named Ancel Keys, but his hypothesis was later disproved. We now know that cholesterol is a normal and necessary part of the human body. (The cholesterol in foods like eggs is necessary for making hormones; it also plays a role in good digestion.) We also now know that the cholesterol in the foods you eat—including eggs—is rarely to blame if you have high cholesterol in your blood; in fact, the less cholesterol you eat, the more your liver will make.

I want you to eat eggs from chickens that are raised humanely and that are able to run free and graze on grass; their eggs are extremely healthy. Be careful about the eggs in the supermarket, though, even organic eggs. They are generally from chickens that are "vegetarian" and "grain fed." The eggs of organic grain-fed chickens don't contain antibiotics, hormones, or chemical residues, which is good. But chickens are not meant to be vegetarians! So look for eggs from chickens that are allowed to range freely outside and eat grass (plus worms and bugs), along with organic grain. You are most likely to get the best free-range eggs from an organic farmer, a neighbor who keeps chickens, a farmers' market, or a natural food store.

Eggs from free-range chickens really are one of nature's perfect foods. They are high in protein (one egg has about 7 g) as well as vitamin B12 (a must for the proper function of the nervous system), vitamin E (a potent antioxidant), choline (a nutrient that supports brain function), and iodine (a trace element your thyroid requires to make hormones). Eggs also contain some vitamin A (critical for immunity and digestion) and vitamin D (see chapter 7 for more information)—two fat-soluble nutrients that are very hard, if not impossible, to come by if you don't eat any animal foods.

Most eggs produced commercially, on the other hand, are very far from perfect. Since they come from chickens that are fed grains, not grass, their fatty acid profile isn't healthful. What's more, the grains they eat often contain pesticides and are from genetically modified crops. The chickens are kept in dismal conditions that promote illness, so they are loaded up with antibiotics in an effort to prevent them from getting sick.

In 1987, the Framingham Heart Study concluded that if you are less than fifty years old, high cholesterol can be a marker for heart disease. If you are over fifty, however, there's no connection between cholesterol levels and your risk of heart disease. In fact, high cholesterol in elderly people is generally associated with good health. A small percentage of people do carry a gene that makes them prone to familial hypercholesterolemia, and these people may need to take cholesterol-lowering drugs. But these drugs are not the answer for everyone else; in fact, they have many negative and dangerous side effects.

Another thing: We've been warned never to eat raw or undercooked eggs because of the potential for salmonella contamination, but it's my understanding that if you choose very fresh eggs from pastured chickens kept in clean conditions, the likelihood you will contract salmonella is very, very low. I've kept my own backyard chickens for years and I eat raw egg yolks without fear; they are a wonderful way to add protein and nutrients to smoothies. Please note, however, that egg whites should not be consumed raw—they contain a substance called avidin that binds to the biotin, a B vitamin, in the yolks and makes it unavailable to your body.

As for cooking eggs, some sources state that you should not eat fried or scrambled eggs (and that you should only boil or poach them) because putting the yolk in direct contact with high heat damages the cholesterol. On the other hand, many health experts believe this simply isn't true and say you should enjoy free-range farm-fresh eggs cooked any way you darn well please, so I do. In their book *The Happiness Diet* (2011), Tyler Graham and

Drew Ramsey suggest pairing eggs with cheese because the vitamin D in the eggs increases the bioavailability of the calcium in the cheese. I don't need an excuse to add cheese to my eggs, but I'll take it.

Eggs are a familiar food in just about every culture in the world, so the ways in which they can be incorporated into recipes are almost infinite. I probably eat at least two eggs pretty much every day; I also use them in dessert recipes. The only reason I can think of not to eat eggs is if you have an egg allergy or sensitivity (recall from chapter 11 that eggs do happen to be a common food sensitivity).

QUICK REVIEW

→ Don't avoid eggs because they are a source of cholesterol; information available to the public regarding cholesterol has been very misleading!

→ Eat farm-fresh, organic eggs from free-range chickens for all the goodness they contain.

→ High quality eggs are a source of omega-3 fats, vitamins A and D, choline, and vitamin B12. If you aren't allergic or sensitive to eggs, you should eat them (cooked any way you like).

SMOKED WILD SALMON AND CRÈME FRAÎCHE OMELET

Serves 1

I adore smoked salmon, and one of my favorite ways to eat it is in this omelet, embellished with my homemade crème fraîche (you'll find the recipe on page 124). This takes just moments to make, yet tastes quite indulgent. Use the highest quality butter, eggs, and smoked salmon (wild, of course) that you can find for the healthiest omelet. Serve it with a salad for a quick and nourishing meal at any time of the day.

2 farm-fresh free-range eggs

1 tbsp crème fraîche, *homemade (page 124) or store-bought; or substitute plain yogurt, good quality cream, or cream cheese*

2 tsp butter, *preferably from pastured cows*

1 oz/30 g wild smoked salmon, *chopped*

2 to 3 tsp minced red onion

1 tsp wild capers *(optional)*

Freshly ground black pepper

1 medium ripe tomato, *sliced, for serving (optional)*

...continued

1 Whisk together the eggs and crème fraîche in a small bowl. The crème fraîche will not blend completely, but this is fine.

2 Heat a small skillet, preferably cast-iron, over medium-high heat. Add the butter. As it melts, use a spoon or metal spatula to move it around, making sure the entire surface of the pan is coated with the butter.

3 Add the egg mixture. Tilt the pan (in several directions, if needed) so that the eggs coat the entire surface. Cook over medium-high heat until the egg in the center of the pan starts to solidify and the edges look slightly brown.

4 Scatter the salmon, red onion, and capers, if using, over half the omelet. Sprinkle with pepper and cook for 20 to 30 seconds more. With a spatula, loosen the side of the omelet without the filling and fold it over the filled half. Continue cooking for another 10 to 20 seconds, and fold the omelet in half again lengthwise, if desired.

5 Remove to a plate and garnish with sliced tomato and more black pepper, if you like.

24 / RECONSIDER MEAT

SOMETIMES PEOPLE LOOK AT ME STRANGELY when I tell them that I eat meat. It's as if I am not supposed to be a carnivore if I am interested in matters of health. I find this somewhat ironic, since the reason I eat meat is *because* of my health.

Meat is a polarizing topic—there is no doubt about that. On one side of the argument, there are those who believe that eating meat is awful for your body, your conscience, and the environment. On the other side, there are folks like me who believe that animals can be raised in a way that's humane and beneficial for the land, and that their meat can be extremely healthy.

I don't like the idea of killing animals, and I can't and won't disconnect myself from the fact that animals do, indeed, need to be killed in order for us to eat meat. But I feel best when there's some meat in my life. This is not going to be true for everyone; if you are a vegetarian and you feel energetic and well without meat, then there may be no reason for you to change the way you eat. Many people can absolutely be healthy vegetarians, especially if they eat high quality eggs and dairy (and maybe a little fish every now and then). If, however, you are a vegetarian, but you do not feel well, then you might want to reconsider meat.

All our ancestors were hunters; people throughout history have sought out and appreciated meat because it has a rich nutritional profile. Meat is a source of protein, iron, phosphorus, B vitamins (including B12, a nutrient that is essential for the nervous system and is only found in animal foods), zinc, and selenium. The meat from cows, lambs, goats, and bison also contains omega-3s and conjugated linoleic acid (CLA, a special fatty acid that appears to have weight-reducing and anticancer properties), but only when that meat is grass fed.

It's crucial to understand that the very best place for cows and other ruminants to be is out on ample pasture. These animals evolved to eat grass and only grass—they get sick when they eat grains. I find it rather magical that with nothing more than grass to work with, their meat and fat can be loaded with the vast array of nutrients I mentioned earlier—and I am incredibly grateful for these foods.

Though I appreciate that cows and other methane-producing animals contribute to greenhouse gases, I believe traditional animal husbandry is a sustainable practice, and I want to support family farms who allow their animals to graze. Sadly, in many parts of the world (including Argentina, where all beef used to be grass fed), the landscape has been radically altered to grow feed—principally soy and corn—for cattle that should be eating grass.

Just as eggs from pastured chickens are completely different (nutritionally speaking) than eggs from their confined, grain-fed counterparts, grass-fed meat is a world away from grain-fed, commercial meat. I would need many pages—or maybe even a whole book—to talk about all that is wrong with modern industrial meat. (For a thorough evaluation of those issues, and an explanation of why even vegetable farms need animals, I recommend the meat chapter in Nina Planck's incredible book *Real Food: What to Eat and Why,* published in 2006.) It goes without saying, however, that I do not want you to eat meat from animals that have not been raised humanely; if you do, you'll be ingesting residues from antibiotics and hormones, not to mention GMOs and pesticides that are in whatever the animals are fed. I also cannot condone the conditions in which the animals are kept.

What about the saturated fat in meat, though? Isn't that going to clog our arteries and cause heart attacks? Well, not exactly. As I mentioned in chapter 19, there has long been a misguided notion that saturated fat contributes to heart disease by doing this *and* by raising our cholesterol, and that's why we've been cautioned not to eat red meat. Like cholesterol, saturated fats aren't all bad. They are important for the structure of all the cells in the body, boost the immune system, and are necessary for the absorption of minerals such as calcium. Saturated fats are also necessary for optimal storage and assimilation of the unsaturated omega-3s. In other words, omega-3 fats are even more effective when they are combined in the diet with some saturated fats.

This is why butter, egg yolks, lard, and duck fat can be perfectly good for you, as long as they are from grass-fed or pastured animals. Lard and duck fat actually contain quite a lot of monounsaturated fat; there is evidence that they lower LDL ("bad") cholesterol and leave HDL ("good") cholesterol alone. (This is great news as far as I am concerned, since piecrust made with lard is seriously fantastic, as are potatoes roasted in duck fat.) I find that many people are still deathly afraid of these fats, especially lard, but keep in mind I am not talking about the highly refined lard you'd find in a typical grocery store. I am talking about lard rendered from the fat

If cholesterol and saturated fats are not to blame for heart disease, what does cause it and how can you prevent it? Current research points to many possible factors, including the overconsumption of refined carbohydrates like wheat and sugar (and the resulting chronically high insulin); a diet high in hydrogenated or trans fats; untreated inflammation in the body; a lack of B vitamins, antioxidants, and omega-3 fats; inadequate exercise; and improperly managed stress. The good news: This book gives you the tools to deal with all of these potential problems, so you can decrease your personal risk.

of pastured pigs. Always remember that when you're eating animal foods, the environment in which the animal was raised has everything to do with whether or not the meat and the fat of that animal will be good for you.

If you eat meat—and I hope after this discussion that you will at least consider making room for a little in your diet—buy it from a local farm or a butcher that sells grass-fed or pastured animal products. Beef, chicken, lamb, pork (yes, even bacon), and other meats can all be part of a healthy diet as long as the animals ate what they were meant to eat (not grains). You can also feel free to eat wild game; more power to you if you hunt it yourself.

A note about grilling meat: Heterocyclic amines (HCA) and polycyclic aromatic hydrocarbons (PAH) are potentially carcinogenic (cancer-causing) chemicals that are associated with grilled foods. You know how the fat from your burger (yes, even a grass-fed one) or your salmon drips down into the fire, and then there's that little flare-up that sends smoke shooting back up? And you know how you get those portions of meat or fish that end up kind of charred? Well, that is how these compounds are created, and it's not a good thing.

Marinating fatty cuts of meat and fish for at least ten minutes (and as long as overnight) before you cook them helps to form a barrier, and cuts down on the carcinogenic chemicals. A good choice for a marinade appears to be one that includes an acidic ingredient, such as vinegar or citrus juice, berries, or cherries; herbs or spices; and some oil. Including tamari (wheat-free fermented soy sauce) in your marinade is also recommended. Eating lots of fruits and vegetables is protective against all cancers, so make sure these are part of your diet, as well.

QUICK REVIEW

➜ Meat can be very nutritious, as long as it is grass fed or pastured. Reconsider meat if you previously avoided it because you believed it to be unhealthy. Buy from a local butcher or a farm that offers grass-fed or pastured animals.

➜ Do not worry about the saturated fat in high quality meat. Saturated fat has many functions in the body. Among other things, it helps you to best utilize the omega-3 fats that you eat.

➜ When grilling fatty cuts of meat (and fish, as well), use an acidic marinade before cooking; this helps to cut down on the potentially carcinogenic chemicals that are associated with grilled foods.

ROASTED CHICKEN AND VEGETABLES

Serves 4

I love this high-heat method for roasting chicken (inspired by chef Thomas Keller), because it's done in less than an hour. This recipe is very adaptable. Sometimes I choose red potatoes, and sometimes I go for sweet potatoes or a combination of the two. Once in a while I fill the pan with chopped winter squash, rutabagas, or turnips instead of potatoes. The only thing I never vary is the garlic (my daughter adores roasted garlic).

Once your roasted chicken is picked over, pack up the carcass and store it in the freezer. When you've got two or three, you can use them to make Homemade Chicken Stock (page 37). Any leftover roast chicken makes a wonderful addition to a salad.

One 3- to 3½-lb/1.4- to 1.6-kg farm-fresh, free-range roasting chicken

2 tbsp butter, *preferably from pastured cows*

Coarse sea salt and freshly ground black pepper

2 sprigs fresh rosemary

1 lemon, *halved*

1½ lb/680 g small red potatoes, *halved, or* **sweet potatoes,** *chopped, or a combination of the two*

2 medium carrots or parsnips, *peeled if not organic and chopped*

6 garlic cloves, *peeled*

1 small onion or 2 shallots, *peeled and chopped*

...continued

1 Preheat the oven to 450°F/230°C.

2 Remove the giblets from the chicken (you can freeze them to add to chicken stock; I usually give them to my dogs). Rinse the chicken very well inside and out. Pat completely dry with a paper towel and place on a cutting board.

3 In a large ovenproof cast-iron skillet, melt the butter. Brush it all over the chicken, and then sprinkle liberally sea salt and black pepper. Stuff the cavity with the rosemary and the lemon halves. If you'd like to truss the chicken, tuck the wings behind the chicken's back and tie the drumsticks together (to be honest, I don't usually bother).

4 Fill the skillet you used to melt the butter with the potatoes, carrots, garlic, and onion. Stir the vegetables around so they're coated with the residual butter left in the skillet. Alternatively, you can melt the butter in a dish in the microwave, brush it over the chicken and drizzle it over the vegetables, and then cook everything in a small roasting pan.

5 Place the chicken on top of the vegetables, breast-side down. Roast for 30 minutes.

6 Wear oven mitts to remove the skillet from the oven (be careful because it will be heavy) and, using sturdy tongs, turn the chicken over. Roast for another 20 to 30 minutes, depending on the size of the chicken, until it is beautifully browned; the juices run clear when the chicken is pierced with a knife; and a thermometer inserted into the inner thigh, but not touching the bone, registers 165°F/75°C.

7 Remove from the oven and allow the chicken to sit in the pan for 5 to 10 minutes before carving. Serve the chicken alongside the vegetables, with the pan juices spooned over all.

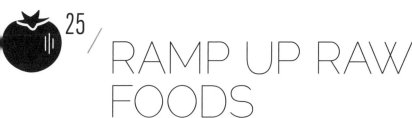

25 / RAMP UP RAW FOODS

DOES IT SEEM STRANGE that I am following the meat chapter with one about raw foods? It shouldn't if you consider that our ancestral diet was made up of large amounts of both. Paleolithic considerations aside, I think everyone should be eating lots of raw foods because they are replete with vitamins, minerals, and live enzymes, which aid digestion and nutrient absorption (and are not, for the most part, present in cooked foods). Raw foods are also high in fiber.

Diets high in raw foods are more nutrient dense than those made up mostly of cooked foods, and eating more raw foods can be a good way to shed some weight and gain more energy. There is also evidence that having lots of raw food in the diet may aid in preventing or healing a number of chronic diseases, including cancer.

How much of your diet do I think should be raw? I am not talking about eating anything close to a 100 percent raw food diet, which is typically a vegan diet, in which nothing is heated over 120°F/48°C. That is a diet that some folks swear by, and it has some positive attributes, but it's very restrictive. As you know from previous chapters, I believe the right types of animal foods support health and should be a part of your diet (unless you avoid eating animal foods for ethical reasons and you feel healthy and energetic). So a good percentage to shoot for would be 30 percent (though I would probably aim higher if I had a health challenge).

Because more and more people are interested in raw foods, you will notice in pretty much any natural food store (and in many other establishments, as well) the availability of items designed for people who follow a raw or close to raw (a.k.a. "high raw") lifestyle. I'm talking about raw energy bars, drinks, crackers, cookies, and cereals. These can be expensive, but they

If you choose to include raw milk, eggs, fish, and meat in your diet, make sure to buy them from trusted sources only. If you are going to prepare a dish with raw meat, it should be of the highest quality, and definitely grass fed or pastured. To be honest, when it comes to fruits, vegetables, and anything else you are going to eat raw (or eat at all, frankly), you should be conscious of the quality, too. Buy the best you can afford (or grow your own), and eat local and organic, if possible. If you can't get your hands on organic ingredients, clean your produce with a wash designed to remove all chemical residues.

definitely make good alternatives to "junkier" options if you're out and about and looking for a snack.

You'll also see a lot of books on the market that are geared toward raw foodies. I have a bunch, and I've learned some cool tips about raw food preparation from them.

Eating more raw foods does not have to be complicated, though; I bet you could easily add more raw fruits and vegetables (or a smoothie or fresh juice) to your meals and snacks. And you can learn how to make a salad that's so awesome that it *is* your meal or snack.

Keep in mind that eating more raw foods doesn't have to be limited to plain old fruits and vegetables. Raw foods you can and should eat more of also include lacto-fermented or cultured fruits and vegetables (more on these in chapter 27); soaked and sprouted raw nuts, seeds, and grains (if you eat them); raw milk and other raw dairy products; raw free-range eggs; and raw wild fish. Beef and lamb have traditionally been consumed raw in some parts of the world, including Europe and the Middle East. Keep in mind that if you have issues with your digestion, you may feel better eating most of your food cooked.

QUICK REVIEW

⇢ Include raw foods in your diet—they are high in fiber, vitamins, minerals, and live enzymes.

⇢ Add a fresh juice or smoothie to your day, or make a meal out of a salad. Other ways to get more raw foods: Eat lacto-fermented or cultured fruits and vegetables (try the Spicy Lacto-Fermented Pickles, page 100); as well as raw nuts, seeds, and soaked and sprouted grains.

⇢ Seek out raw milk and cheese, add raw free-range egg yolks to smoothies, and experiment with raw wild fish and even raw grass-fed meat. (Buy from a trusted source.)

BLENDED RAW TOMATO-BASIL SOUP

Serves 2

While I like traditional cooked tomato soup as much as the next person, I think this raw tomato soup is even better, especially when you make it with seasonal organic tomatoes. It's a bit like gazpacho, but with a pared-down list of ingredients.

I grow a very large variety of heirloom tomatoes in my garden, so I like to mix them in a range of colors in this soup. A combination of red and yellow tomatoes yields a soup that looks remarkably similar to a cream-based one. Basil and tomatoes get along fabulously, both in the garden and in recipes, so I grow lots of basil, too.

This makes a nice light lunch with a fried egg on top.

4 medium tomatoes, preferably heirloom varieties in season, *cored and quartered*

4 olive oil–packed sun-dried tomatoes *(optional)*

1 tbsp avocado oil or olive oil

Handful of fresh basil leaves, *plus more (optional) for garnish*

¼ tsp fine sea salt, or to taste

Diced avocado for garnish *(optional)*

Pinch of smoked paprika for garnish *(optional)*

1 Place both kinds of tomatoes, the avocado oil, basil, and salt in a blender and blend until fairly smooth (I personally prefer the soup with some texture). Pour into bowls and garnish with the diced avocado, fresh basil, and smoked paprika, if desired.

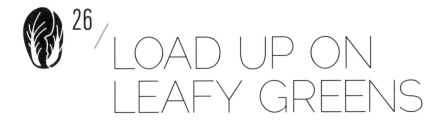

26 / LOAD UP ON LEAFY GREENS

IN THE PREVIOUS CHAPTER, I shared the benefits of raw foods. In this one, I want to put the spotlight on the very healthful leafy greens.

Leafy greens are low in calories and carbohydrates, yet extremely high in nutrients; they contain significant amounts of vitamins A, B2, C, E, and K, as well as folic acid and fiber. They're also full of beneficial phytochemicals and carotenoids, which are protective against cancer. Finally, leafy greens have a healthy alkalizing effect on the body due to their mineral content (notably calcium, magnesium, potassium, and iron).

Not sure what I mean by leafy greens? I am talking about arugula, beet greens, bok choy (and other Asian greens, such as tatsoi and mizuna), broccoli rabe, members of the cabbage family (including broccoli and kohlrabi, which, while not technically leafy, are still green and healthy), cilantro and parsley (although herbs, these can also be considered leafy greens), chicory, collard greens, endive, escarole, frisée, kale (all varieties), mixed greens (mesclun), mustard greens, radicchio, romaine lettuce, sorrel, spinach, Swiss chard (red, green, and rainbow), turnip greens, watercress, and wild greens (such as chickweed, dandelion, lamb's-quarters, nettles, and purslane).

I wish I could simply say "Okay, go eat as much as you can of the greens mentioned above" and be done with it. But it's not that quite that simple.

First of all, the cruciferous vegetables (those in the Brassica genus of plants) are goitrogenic, meaning they can suppress thyroid function (because they block iodine absorption) when they are eaten to excess in their raw form. Cruciferous vegetables include arugula, bok choy, broccoli, Brussels sprouts, cabbage, collard greens, kohlrabi, kale, and watercress. They are loaded with cancer-fighting nutrients, but you should eat them cooked as well as raw.

Does that mean you should never eat cabbage or kale salads? No. It just means you shouldn't live on them, and if you already have thyroid issues, you should eat them raw even more sparingly. I like raw kale salads a lot, but I mostly eat kale that's been cooked. As for cabbage, it's probably healthiest when it's been transformed into sauerkraut or kimchi because it will be at its most digestible and contain the most nutrients.

The second reason it's not safe to eat raw greens with abandon is that some of them—including beet greens, Swiss chard, spinach, parsley, purslane, and lamb's-quarters—contain high amounts of oxalic acid. And oxalic acid inhibits mineral absorption (particularly calcium and iron), which is a real bummer, since one of the main reasons many of us eat these greens is because of the minerals. Oxalic acid may also contribute to kidney stones. Cooking reduces the oxalic acid in these veggies, so again, the main concern is if you eat large amounts of them raw.

It's interesting to note that while some greens have a bitter taste that many consider a turnoff, this bitterness is one of the reasons they are so good for you. Bitter foods stimulate the digestive organs to produce hydrochloric acid. As a result, they can help boost a sluggish appetite, aid in fat and protein absorption, relieve gas and constipation, and help with heartburn. (Many who suffer from heartburn mistakenly assume they have too much acid, but the problem is more often a hydrochloric acid *deficiency*.) So if you have trouble with your digestion, consider starting each meal with a salad of bitter greens (such as dandelion greens, chicory, radicchio, or a combination) dressed with some lemon juice (the acid in the lemon juice helps you absorb the iron in the greens). Bitter herbal formulas taken with meals can also help, and have long been popular in Europe (think Swedish bitters).

QUICK REVIEW

⇢ Leafy greens are nutrient powerhouses. Enjoy some of them raw (a small amount can be blended into smoothies), some in cooked form, and some lacto-fermented.

⇢ Raw greens in the cruciferous family can block iodine absorption and suppress the thyroid gland; other raw greens contain high amounts of oxalic acid. Make sure to eat a wide variety of greens, including the very nutritional ones.

⇢ A small salad of bitter greens at the beginning of a meal is particularly good for digestion.

MIXED GREEN SALAD with APPLE, GOAT CHEESE, and SOFT-BOILED EGGS

Serves 1 or 2

This salad makes the perfect lunch for one person, or it can be divided into two smaller dinner salads to serve along with a main dish. Feel free to change it up by using different greens or another cheese (I love it with small chunks of raw ched-dar). The nuts are optional but add welcome crunch and additional nutrients. Pears can stand in for the apples, of course, and a handful of fresh pomegranate seeds on top adds a pretty and delicious touch.

SALAD

2 handfuls of mixed baby greens (mesclun)

Handful of shredded kale, *preferably Tuscan kale, tough stems removed*

Handful of chopped sorrel or young arugula, *or use additional baby greens or kale*

1 small crunchy apple, *peeled if not organic, and chopped (or slice the apple instead for an elegant presentation)*

2 to 3 tbsp crumbled goat cheese

½ cup/55 g walnuts or pecans *(optional)*

Pinch of coarse sea salt and freshly ground black pepper

2 farm-fresh free-range eggs

DRESSING

2 tbsp toasted walnut oil or olive oil

1 tbsp balsamic vinegar or fresh lemon juice

1½ tsp pure maple syrup

1 tsp minced shallot

Coarse sea salt and freshly ground black pepper

1 To make the salad: Toss the baby greens, kale, and sorrel together in a medium bowl. Add the apple, goat cheese, and nuts, if desired. Season with salt and black pepper.

2 Put the eggs in a small pot of cold water to cover and bring to a simmer. Cook for exactly 5 minutes (set a timer) from the time the water starts to simmer. Remove the eggs from the pan with a slotted spoon and rinse under cold water. Carefully remove the shells from the eggs, cut in half, and set aside.

3 To make the dressing: Whisk the oil, vinegar, maple syrup, and shallot together in a small bowl. Taste and season lightly with salt and black pepper.

4 To serve, pour the dressing over the salad. Add the eggs and use two forks to gently toss everything together.

27 / GET SOME CULTURE

THOUGH I'VE LONG KNOWN THAT CULTURED FOODS like yogurt are good for you, I did not completely understand why until I read the book *Nourishing Traditions*, which I highly recommend. Author Sally Fallon points out that naturally cultured foods and drinks were prevalent in the diets of our ancestors, yet they're scarcely consumed by most people today.

Fallon proposes that we are doing our bodies a great disservice by ignoring traditionally cultured foods. You see, cultured foods are teeming with vitamins, live enzymes, and natural probiotics—bacteria that are helpful for reducing the amount of harmful organisms in the intestines. Cultured foods foster a healthy digestive environment, and contribute to optimal wellness overall.

Bacteria known as lactobacilli convert sugars and starches into lactic acid. The presence of lots of lactic acid results in a food that's exceptionally nutritious and much less prone to spoilage. Before there was refrigeration and before foods were canned to extend their shelf life, they were naturally preserved in small batches using the lacto-fermentation method.

Dairy products like yogurt, kefir, and crème fraîche (and also many cheeses); miso (a lacto-fermented soybean paste); kombucha (a lacto-fermented beverage made from tea); and vegetable preparations such as kimchi, lacto-fermented pickles, and sauerkraut are all examples of cultured foods.

Nowadays, most pickles, sauerkraut, and many brands of yogurt available at the supermarket are not lacto-fermented: they're made with vinegar and sugar, and they're pasteurized (which kills off the enzymes). If you want to take advantage of the health benefits these foods have traditionally offered, you must seek out versions with live cultures.

Cultured foods (and particularly cultured vegetables) are good for everyone, but they are particularly useful if your digestion is poor or your immune system is weak (this can manifest itself as environmental allergies, food sensitivities, or catching frequent colds). Eating cultured foods is also suggested if you're struggling to balance your blood sugar, want to lose weight, get frequent yeast infections, or are pregnant. I try to include at least one serving of lacto-fermented foods in my diet every day, but I eat much more when I have any sort of stomach issue going on or on the rare occasion that I have to take antibiotics.

You can purchase high quality versions of cultured foods at natural food stores, but I think knowing how to make your own is a good skill to have (plus you'll save money). This is why I am giving you recipes for Spicy Lacto-Fermented Pickles (page 100), Homemade Yogurt (page 39), and Do-It-Yourself Crème Fraîche (page 124).

QUICK REVIEW

→ Cultured foods are fantastic for the body. You should eat them every day.

→ Dairy products like yogurt, kefir, and crème fraîche (and many cheeses); the soybean paste miso; the beverage kombucha; and vegetable preparations like kimchi, lacto-fermented pickles, and sauerkraut are all cultured foods.

→ Cultured vegetables are particularly beneficial, since they're high in nutrients and fiber; you can add them to all sorts of dishes as condiments.

Did you know that your digestive system and your immune system are intimately linked? About 75 percent of your immune system's cells reside in your digestive tract; if your digestive system isn't functioning optimally, your health as a whole will suffer. Cultured foods are a great source of the "good bacteria" that your digestive system requires in order to run smoothly.

Our digestive systems are incredibly complex and unbelievably fragile; it's very important to make sure they stay in good shape. In addition to relaxing when you eat and including lacto-fermented foods in your diet, there are many other things you can do to foster optimal digestion. As I mentioned in the previous chapter, bitter herbs and greens are excellent. I also recommend soaking your grains before you cook them. Eating protein foods like eggs and dairy products in their full-fat state is important, because the fats aid digestion. Cooking with stocks that are rich in natural gelatin, such as Homemade Chicken Stock (page 37) helps, too. There are also supplements, including encapsulated probiotics, that can aid in the support and healing of the digestive tract; speak to your natural health care practitioner if you think you might benefit from these.

SPICY LACTO-FERMENTED PICKLES

*Makes enough to fill
a 1-qt/960-ml jar*

*According to traditional foods expert Sally Fallon, an ambient temperature of
72°F/22°C is ideal for making lacto-fermented vegetables. At this temperature, the
process should take 2 to 4 days (if your kitchen is cooler, it will take longer, and
if it's warmer, things will speed up). These pickles are a little bit sweet and pack
quite a bit of heat; I adore them and snack on them frequently. For a more classic
pickle, see the following variation.*

**5 or 6 pickling (Kirby) cucumbers,
or 6 or 7 small Persian cucumbers
(about 1 lb/455 g),** *ends trimmed off,
and cut into 1-in/2.5-cm pieces*

1 tbsp fine sea salt

**1 tbsp all-natural Thai fish sauce or
wheat-free tamari**

1 tbsp pure maple syrup

1 jalapeño pepper, *thinly sliced*

1 tbsp minced garlic

1 tbsp minced ginger

EQUIPMENT

**One 1-qt/960-ml glass canning
jar with a screw-top lid,** *metal or
BPA-free plastic*

1 Clean the glass jar and lid in hot, soapy water, or use the hottest setting on your dishwasher.

2 Combine the cucumbers with the salt, fish sauce, maple syrup, jalapeño, garlic, and ginger in a medium bowl, then transfer everything to the glass jar. If a few of the cucumber pieces don't fit, that's fine; you can just eat them.

3 Add enough filtered water so the liquid covers the cucumbers. Be sure to leave 1 in/2.5 cm of room at the top of the jar before capping tightly with the lid. (If you don't leave enough room, liquid may seep out of your jar as the pickles ferment.)

4 Allow your pickles to sit at room temperature for 2 to 4 days. You'll know they're done when the brine begins to bubble; do not worry if the brine is a bit cloudy—this is completely normal. Enjoy right away, or store in the refrigerator, where the pickles will keep for at least 2 to 3 weeks; the heat from the jalapeños will mellow a bit as they sit in the brine.

VARIATION

For a more classic pickle, omit everything but the cucumbers and salt. Cut the cucumbers into spears instead. Add another tbsp of salt, 5 peeled cloves of garlic and 10 peppercorns, and 2 or 3 sprigs of fresh dill. The directions are otherwise the same.

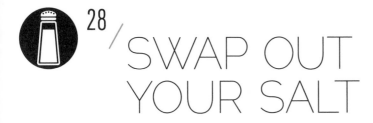

28 / SWAP OUT YOUR SALT

POOR SALT; it gets such a bad rap. Let's talk about why you should not necessarily restrict the salt in your diet, and why the type of salt you choose to consume really makes all the difference in how salt affects you.

Salt is vital; in his book *Your Body's Many Cries for Water* (1995), author Dr. F. Batmanghelidj notes, "Oxygen, water, salt, and potassium rank as the primary elements for the survival of the human body." Salt is 40 percent sodium and 60 percent chloride by weight. It performs many jobs: Salt maintains the fluid volume in our blood, regulates the acidity in our cells, and must be present for proper nerve and muscle function. In addition, the enzymes that break down the complex carbohydrates we eat depend on sodium, while chloride is necessary for the formation of hydrochloric acid (which we need in ample amounts for optimal digestion).

Salt in some form has always been part of the human diet, yet it's been demonized in the modern mainstream nutritional literature because of the supposed connection between a high-salt diet and high blood pressure (which increases your risk of heart disease and stroke). While it is true that some individuals are salt sensitive and will experience a rise in blood pressure when they consume salt, this is not the case for everyone. In fact, the majority of people are likely to end up with problems from overly restricting salt because a salt deficiency can cause insulin resistance, osteoporosis, cancer, and, ironically, heart failure.

I am going to ask you to recall the discussion about sugar back in chapter 14 for a moment. Remember how I talked about the fact that refined white sugar was bad for you, but that less processed types of sugar are okay? The situation with salt is very similar. Refined salt (a.k.a. table salt) is definitely not good for you, and most people do consume way too much. Table salt has had all its naturally occurring minerals stripped away; it's heavily processed, and it contains chemical additives. This type of salt is found in all packaged and processed foods, and it's what most people add to their food when they cook at home or eat out. Refined salt is not the type of salt your body needs. Just as your body prefers natural foods instead of processed ones, your body functions best when you consume natural, not processed, salt.

If you go to the grocery store these days, you're likely to find a dizzying array of salts for sale. In addition to table salt, you'll find kosher salt, sea salts, and maybe other types of "gourmet" salts, as well. There are so many choices; it can be hard to know what kind of salt to buy. Many people, particularly chefs and home-cooking enthusiasts, have taken to using kosher salt because its larger crystals make it easy to add to foods and because it has a pure salty flavor (it's just salt with no additives). While I do sometimes use kosher salt in my kitchen, the salt I reach for most of the time is sea salt. I have a few different kinds in my pantry, including Himalayan crystal salt, Celtic sea salt, French *fleur de sel*, and several varieties of Hawaiian sea salts.

Okay, you may be thinking, but what about iodine? It's added to table salt for a good reason, right? If we don't eat table salt, will we get enough?

Iodine is a water-soluble trace element required by the thyroid gland to make hormones. If you don't get enough iodine, you can end up with an enlarged thyroid gland (a.k.a. goiter). Iodine has been added to table salt in the United States since the 1920s as a preventative measure against this condition. An iodine deficiency can also cause other thyroid problems, which can affect your health in many negative ways. An iodine deficiency during pregnancy can be very serious (it stunts both mental and physical growth in the fetus). It is also linked to heart disease, prostate cancer, fibrocystic breasts, and breast cancer.

The amount of iodine present in foods is dependent upon the soil in which they're grown, or the body of water from which they're harvested. Indeed, foods

If you frequently experience strong cravings for salty foods, please consider the possibility that you've got too much going on in your life. Being overworked or overly busy or worrying a lot puts a lot of stress on your adrenal glands, and they can get burned out. People with depleted adrenal glands generally have very low blood pressure and thus the desire to eat salty foods. Including moderate amounts of the healthful sea salts in your diet will help you nourish your adrenal glands, and so will getting adequate rest, making time for relaxation, and learning how to manage your stress (go back to chapter 5 if you need a stress-management refresher).

from the sea—such as fish, seafood, and seaweed—are among the best sources of iodine. Vegetables can also contain iodine, as can eggs, meat, and dairy products (as long as the animals are grazed on grass grown in iodine-rich soil). You don't need iodine in large amounts; if you eat a varied diet that contains land and sea animals as well as land and sea plant foods, you are probably getting enough. If you only eat plant foods, then you're more at risk for an iodine deficiency.

It's important to understand that even if you're taking in enough iodine, if you are also eating a lot of the goitrogenic foods mentioned in chapter 26, they can interfere with your thyroid's ability to utilize the iodine. This is why it's important to cut back on goitrogens in their raw form if you have any thyroid issues at all; it's also important to limit soy foods (soy is another goitrogen) if that's the case. If you have issues with your thyroid, speak to your doctor to determine how best to support this important gland (and to see if you might need supplemental iodine).

QUICK REVIEW

→ Salt isn't unhealthy for most people (in fact, it is necessary for proper functioning of the body). Swap out your table salt for a natural sea salt that's high in minerals and trace elements. There are many to choose from: Celtic sea salt, in particular, has many therapeutic properties.

→ When you switch your iodized salt for sea salt, make sure you take in enough iodine to keep your thyroid gland healthy (and watch out for goitrogenic foods, including raw cruciferous vegetables, because they interfere with iodine absorption).

→ Eat fish and seafood (review chapter 22 for the healthiest varieties), seaweeds, and a variety of plant and pastured animal foods to ensure you get enough iodine.

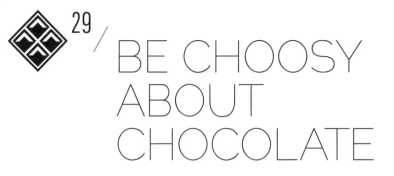

29

BE CHOOSY ABOUT CHOCOLATE

CHOCOLATE IS UNIVERSALLY ADORED, and I'm well aware that I'd be extremely unpopular if I told you that you shouldn't eat it. Good thing I don't have to do that; eating chocolate can mesh with a healthy lifestyle—*the key is to choose the right kind of chocolate.*

Chocolate is made from the cacao (a.k.a. cocoa) bean. These grow on the *Theobroma cacao* tree, which is native to tropical areas in South America (though nowadays the trees are cultivated in other regions, including Africa's Ivory Coast). Long ago, cocoa beans were crushed and made into a savory drink, which was spiced with chile peppers. This beverage is said to have been a favorite of Aztec and Mayan royalty, who believed that drinking it conferred spiritual wisdom as well as vitality. A type of sweetened drinking chocolate was introduced to Europe in the seventeenth century and became very popular among the upper classes.

Cocoa beans have a lot of positive attributes: They are high in minerals, particularly magnesium, and many health experts believe the intense chocolate cravings some people (including women with PMS) experience are driven by a magnesium deficiency. Cocoa beans are also high in natural fats, including a unique saturated fat called stearic acid, which is very stable and appears to have no effect on cholesterol. And the beans contain antioxidants, which are reputed to protect the entire cardiovascular system and lower the risk of heart disease. You may also recall from chapter 7 that consumption of the antioxidants (a.k.a. flavonoids) in cocoa is associated with a decreased risk of getting sunburned. Consumption of cocoa increases certain neurotransmitters (brain chemicals) that positively affect our moods, as well.

This all sounds great, but cocoa beans generally go through such extensive processing that there's very little actual cocoa present in most chocolate;

there is a lot of sugar, unhealthy hydrogenated oils, emulsifiers, and chemical additives, though! That's why the majority of the chocolate that's out there isn't very good for you.

The best chocolate to eat—the chocolate that's actually beneficial to your health—is 70 percent (or more) dark chocolate. I'd also opt for chocolate that's organic (nonorganic may contain pesticides and even lead). A final word: To make sure you avoid buying chocolate that's cultivated by slave labor from third world countries, you'll want to choose chocolate that is fair-trade certified.

You are most likely to find fair-trade organic dark chocolate in a natural food store or artisan chocolate shop. A well-stocked supermarket may carry some brands of high quality chocolate, as well, but most of the chocolate in the grocery store is definitely not healthy.

If you are accustomed to eating milk chocolate, you may find dark chocolate to be an acquired taste. It took some getting used to for me, but I now find dark chocolate to be one of life's greatest pleasures. Because it still contains some sugar, dark chocolate is best for you when consumed in moderation— no surprise there, right? I find that just a square or two from a high quality dark chocolate bar hits the spot.

Another type of healthy chocolate you might want to try is raw chocolate, which is generally sold in powder form or as cacao nibs. The nibs are the raw (unroasted) cocoa bean without the skin, and can be purchased at natural food stores and online. I find these to be extremely bitter, but an interesting addition to smoothies and some desserts. I use raw cacao powder as an alternative to cocoa powder all the time.

QUICK REVIEW

⇨ Eating chocolate can mesh with a healthy lifestyle.

⇨ Opt for chocolate that is organic, fair-trade, low-sugar, and at least 70 percent dark in order to take advantage of its potential health benefits.

⇨ Raw cacao powder and cacao nibs are incredibly nutrient dense, as well, so feel free to experiment with these; they make a great addition to smoothies and desserts.

GRAIN-FREE, FAIR-TRADE CHOCOLATE CHIP COOKIES

Makes about twenty 2-in/5-cm cookies

If you told me chocolate chip cookies were the only dessert I could have for the rest of my life, I'd be totally fine with that; I adore them that much. I came up with this nutrient-dense version to replace the standard chocolate chippers I previously relied on. Happily, my family loved them. These cookies contain protein and healthy fats, but don't go overboard with them—they are meant to be a treat! Although you can use another unrefined sugar, I strongly recommend the coconut sugar; it really makes these cookies delicious.

Blanched almond flour is available from Bob's Red Mill at natural food stores and online.

½ cup/30 g unsweetened shredded coconut

1½ cups/120 g finely ground blanched almond flour

¼ cup/30 g coconut flour

½ tsp baking soda

½ tsp fine sea salt

½ cup/115 g butter, *preferably from pastured cows, at room temperature*

1 cup/150 g coconut sugar, or 1 cup/200 g granulated sugar

1 farm-fresh, free-range egg

1 tsp pure vanilla extract

1 cup/170 g fair-trade dark chocolate chips

...continued

1 Preheat the oven to 325°F/165°C. Line two baking sheets with parchment paper or silicone baking mats.

2 Spread out the coconut on one of the baking sheets and toast in the oven until light brown and fragrant, about 5 minutes, but start watching after 4 minutes so it doesn't burn. Set aside to cool for several minutes. Increase the oven temperature to 350°F/180°C.

3 Using a wire whisk or a fork, mix together the toasted coconut, almond flour, coconut flour, baking soda, and salt in a medium bowl.

4 Using a stand mixer fitted with a paddle attachment or a handheld electric mixer, cream the butter and sugar on low speed until smooth, about 3 minutes. Scrape down the sides of the bowl and the paddle. Add the egg and vanilla and mix until blended.

5 Add the almond flour mixture and beat until just incorporated. Briefly beat in the chocolate chips. Cover the dough and refrigerate for at least 30 minutes (and up to 2 days) before baking.

6 Spoon rounded teaspoons of the dough onto the baking sheets approximately 2 in/5 cm apart.

7 Bake for 15 to 18 minutes, or until the cookies are starting to brown around the edges but still look slightly underdone in the center (they'll continue to cook a bit after you take them out of the oven).

8 Remove the cookies from the oven. Allow them to rest for 1 to 2 minutes on the baking sheets, and then, using a spatula, carefully transfer to a cooling rack. (If you transfer them too soon, they're likely to crumble.) Wait a few more minutes before serving or until completely cooled before storing in an airtight container. The cookies should keep for 4 to 5 days.

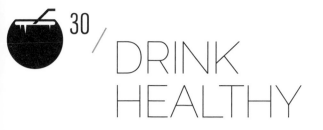

30 / DRINK HEALTHY

BY THIS POINT IN THE BOOK you have learned so much about nutrition and what to eat; I hope integrating the changes is going well and that you are feeling great. Now let's make sure you're not undermining your healthy food choices by reaching for less-than-ideal drinks.

You already know that water should make up a large percentage of the fluid you take in (for a review, see chapter 3). In addition to water, you should feel free to drink homemade vegetable or fruit juices (I'll talk more about juicing in the next chapter). What about juice that's not homemade? I do keep store-bought organic juice in the house, but we don't drink juice straight. Even if there's no added sugar, juice is very sweet, so it's best diluted with still or sparkling water. Look for juices made from fruits that are exceptionally nutritious, such as cherry or pomegranate.

Coconut water is another good choice; it's high in minerals and is a great alternative to sports drinks for replacing electrolytes after vigorous exercise (commercial sports drinks generally contain high-fructose corn syrup, so it's best to avoid them). Make sure to look for high quality brands of coconut water that don't contain sugar or additives.

Nondairy milks (including soy, rice, almond, and hemp milk) have become quite popular and are widely available. I personally gave up drinking soy milk many years ago because it is very processed and there's evidence it can disrupt your hormones (I've never let my kids drink it, either). Rice milk and the others are all right. My main concern is that they are quite sweet and high in carbohydrates, and they are also fairly processed. So I'd suggest consuming them in small quantities. I also like homemade nut milks, which are easy to prepare (see Walnut Milk, page 112).

Dairy milk is a good source of protein and calcium, but I avoid commercially produced milk. In fact, I drink raw whole milk, which is high in enzymes and naturally healthy fats. If you can't find or simply wouldn't consider drinking raw milk, the next best type of milk is pasteurized, unhomogenized whole milk. Why whole milk? Because the fat in it is necessary for the assimilation of the fat-soluble nutrients milk contains. Dairy is a pretty controversial topic, which I talk more about in chapter 33.

Kombucha is a naturally cultured drink high in probiotics and B vitamins. Buy it at a natural food store or, better yet, learn how to make your own. Kombucha is wonderful for enhancing digestion and immunity, and some people claim it boosts their energy, as well. This is what I reach for when I am craving the fizziness of soda but want a healthier option. Along the same lines are homemade or store-bought naturally fermented soft drinks. These are much better for you than sodas filled with high-fructose corn syrup and chemicals, and make a nice treat every now and then.

If you want another alternative to soda, look for the naturally sweetened soda brands that contain absolutely no high-fructose corn syrup (for example, naturally sweetened ginger and root beers). Fruit-flavored sodas are also very tasty, and children usually love them. Read the labels, though, and be aware that these are still high in sugar and carbohydrates, so you shouldn't go overboard with them.

As for coffee and black tea, organic, fair-trade brews are best. Drink them in moderation, because they contain caffeine (which is not healthy in large amounts). I will talk more about these in chapter 35.

Green tea has less caffeine than coffee and black tea and is a great source of antioxidants, which support the immune system. It appears to help with weight loss and weight maintenance, as well. I enjoy green tea frequently. Yerba maté is a healthy herbal drink made from the leaves of a tree that grows in the South American rain forests; it has a little caffeine but is high in nutrients, too.

All-natural coffee substitutes are grain or herb based. Some are made from roasted barley (not appropriate if you eat gluten or grain free) and chicory. Herbal coffee substitutes are high in antioxidants and can be brewed just like coffee.

Organic herbal tea that does not contain caffeine can be warming and comforting at any time of the day. Mint and chamomile are both good choices after a meal, as they promote good digestion. Many herbal teas have so much flavor that they need little sweetening, but a bit of raw honey may be added, if desired.

Another healthy drink to consider is warm chicken or vegetable stock. You can add a little miso or coconut milk (or both) for added benefits. I always drink homemade stock when I am not feeling well—it's a natural immune booster (see page 37 for my recipe). Occasionally I also like to drink a little apple cider vinegar or lemon juice mixed with warm water and a bit of maple syrup or raw honey; it feels very cleansing to me.

QUICK REVIEW

→ Enhance your good diet with drinks that support health.

→ There are many healthy drinks to choose from in addition to water.

→ Healthy drinks include (but are not limited to) juices, real-food smoothies, high quality organic dairy milk, homemade nut milks, kombucha, herbal teas, moderate amounts of organic fair-trade coffee and black tea, green tea, and natural sodas.

WALNUT MILK

Makes 4 cups/960 ml

Though I personally drink organic raw cow's milk, it is sometimes wise to avoid milk. (If you are sensitive to dairy, drinking milk will detract from, rather than enhance, your health.) Nut milks are a nutritious option, and any type of raw nuts (or seeds) can be used to make them. Almond milk is a classic, but delicious milks can be made from pecans, Brazil nuts, cashews, sunflower seeds, pumpkin seeds, and more. This recipe features walnuts, which are high in alpha-linolenic acid (ALA, one of the fatty acids in the omega-3 family).

This makes a good base for a smoothie; you can also serve it with breakfast, or have it plain as a refreshing drink at any time of the day. Nut milks hold up fine if you warm them gently, and I've used them to make hot chocolate. If you don't have the time or inclination to soak the nuts or seeds, you can use about ½ cup/125 g of a nut or seed butter instead. A nut milk bag will come in handy for this recipe (they're available at natural food stores and on Amazon).

1¼ cup/140 g walnuts, *soaked overnight in enough water to cover the nuts by 1 in/2.5 cm*

4 cups/960 ml water

1 to 2 tbsp pure maple syrup

1 tsp pure vanilla extract

Pinch of fine sea salt

1 Drain the walnuts and rinse thoroughly. Combine with the water in a blender and blend for several minutes. You want the nuts to be thoroughly pulverized.

2 Pour through a nut milk bag or a strainer lined with several layers of cheesecloth to strain out the nut pulp (I compost mine). Return the strained liquid to the blender and add the maple syrup, vanilla, and salt. Blend until thoroughly combined. Drink immediately. Any leftover milk will keep in the refrigerator for 3 to 4 days (shake well before serving).

VARIATIONS

Go ahead and play around with the ingredient amounts in this recipe until you get it just the way you like it: Use fewer nuts and add some banana or pitted dates or dried figs (soaked in water for at least 10 minutes to soften them) for a sweeter drink. Or add more nuts and less water for a creamier one. You could also add some ground cinnamon (or another spice) or fair-trade cocoa powder (or raw cacao powder), or use a different (or additional) sweetener.

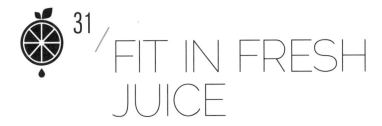

31 / FIT IN FRESH JUICE

I HAVE BEEN DRINKING FRESH JUICE ON AND OFF for about twenty years. I started when I was recovering from my disordered eating and related health problems.

At first, I would buy juice from a juice bar or health food store. I was mostly drinking carrot juice at that point, and after the palms of my hands and the soles of my feet turned orange from the excess beta-carotene, I figured I should branch out and try juicing other vegetables!

I decided to get my own juicer and got more creative with my recipes, but I hated cleaning the juicer. Eventually I stopped making juice and gave the juicer away to a friend. This pattern repeated itself a few more times through the years. I'd get super into juicing—I even did a ten-day juice fast in Hawaii once—and then my enthusiasm would die. I have owned and subsequently given away at least four juicers as a result.

A few years ago, my husband and I started drinking juice again. We soon realized we were spending way too much money at our favorite local juice joint, so we decided to purchase a juicer once more and commit ourselves to drinking only juice made at home. We've sort of stuck to this plan, though sometimes months go by and there's no juicing.

I could go on and on about why juicing is good for you, but I'll try to keep it simple: Fresh juice is a raw, live food that's high in enzymes, and it's absolutely brimming with nutrients that are well absorbed by the body. The juicer does all the work of breaking down the fruits and veggies for you, so juicing is excellent for anyone with any sort of digestive issue. Juicing fruits and vegetables is a wonderful way to increase the amount of nutrients from raw foods in your diet, and fresh juice is super high in minerals that can be used by the body to reduce inflammation and heal numerous ailments. Juicing helps the body rid itself of toxins, so it can be a valuable addition to a weight loss program; many juicing aficionados also believe it improves the condition of your skin and hair.

Be aware that even though fresh juice is fabulous for you, it does not have any fiber. So please don't give up on eating your fruits and veggies whole. Also, as you get into juicing, it's best to juice other vegetables besides carrots (they're high in natural sugar and you might turn orange like I did), or fruit, and as always, be aware of not juicing too many of the goitrogenic greens. Balance is key! Organic produce is recommended for juicing; if you can't buy organic, make sure to wash your fruits and veggies with an all-natural produce rinse to remove any pesticides or other chemical residues.

Fresh juice should be consumed right after you make it (store-bought packaged juices honestly don't have a lot of value in terms of nutrients and healing properties). To optimize digestion, it's best to drink fresh juice twenty to thirty minutes before a meal, and it's best not to guzzle the juice down, but rather to drink it slowly, and sort of "chew" every mouthful.

Yes, it's a bit of a pain to clean the juicer. But think about how much good you are doing your body by incorporating the practice of juicing into your life.

QUICK REVIEW

→ Drinking fresh juice is an excellent way to get more raw foods into your diet; juices are extremely high in nutrients and are very cleansing and healing to the body.

→ Don't drink only carrot juice; many vegetables can be juiced, so experiment to find the blends that you enjoy and that make you feel well.

→ Fresh juice is best when prepared with organic ingredients and consumed right after it's made, preferably twenty to thirty minutes before you have a meal.

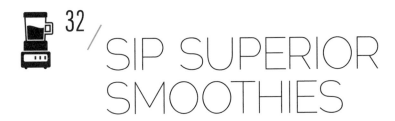

32 / SIP SUPERIOR SMOOTHIES

I LOVE SMOOTHIES, and I'm pretty sure many of you feel the same way. Often referred to as healthy fast food, smoothies are popular because they can be blended in a hurry, and make a quick and tasty breakfast or snack. Smoothies are also infinitely adaptable and, like fresh juices, they are a great way to increase the amount of raw food in your diet.

Some people don't understand how smoothies differ from juices, though, so let's clear that up right away. A fresh juice is a drink made out of a vegetable or fruit in a juicer. Juices are high in enzymes and nutrients, but contain no insoluble fiber (the juicer spits out the fiber). Smoothies are different; they are made in a blender, not a juicer, so they contain fiber. Smoothies can be made with fresh fruits and veggies, such as leafy greens, and you can add lots of other things to smoothies, too. Some of these additions are healthy and some are not; if you make a smoothie with frozen yogurt, store-bought juice, and a bit of fruit, it won't be terribly good for you. A smoothie like that is super-high in sugar without a lot of nutrients.

So let's focus on how to make a truly healthy smoothie—one that's superior in terms of nutrition and taste. First, let's talk about the blender. A high-speed blender (such as a Vitamix or a Blendtec) allows you to incorporate healthy frozen fruits and ice into your smoothies and blend them with ease, giving you a drink with a pleasing creamy consistency. If you're adding greens to your smoothies, a high-speed blender will break them down and blend them into your smoothie completely. I don't think a day goes by when I don't use my high-speed blender, but if you're not ready to invest in one of these, a regular blender can work just fine for smoothies, especially if you only drink them on occasion.

One you've got your blender, the next thing you'll need for a healthy smoothie is some fruit. Some suggestions for fruits to use: bananas, berries (strawberries, blueberries, blackberries, raspberries), peaches, mangoes, papayas, and pineapple. You can use fresh or frozen fruit. Frozen fruit is very convenient, because you can keep it stored in your freezer at all times. It also makes a thicker, creamier smoothie than fresh fruit. Feel free to use a combination of fruits, some fresh and some frozen.

I recommend buying a bunch of different fruits the next time you are at the store. That way you can experiment and come up with your own favorite healthy smoothie recipes. In my freezer, I try to keep large bags of frozen blueberries, raspberries, strawberries, mangoes, and peaches on hand at all times. I also buy lots of bananas, peel them, cut them in half, and store them in BPA-free plastic bags in the freezer. Keep your eyes peeled for deals on overripe bananas, because they're perfect for freezing to use in smoothies. Organic fruits are preferable, but they can be very expensive, especially in the winter. Load up on organic fruit when it's on sale, if possible, and freeze your own fruit when it's in season and locally available.

Once you've decided on your fruits, consider adding some greens. Leafy greens are low in carbohydrates and are very high in vitamins and minerals. They will also balance out the natural sugar of the fruit, which can be considerable. Good choices for mild greens that you probably won't taste in your smoothie include chopped romaine lettuce, a small head of baby bok choy, or a few handfuls of baby spinach or arugula. Again, one of the advantages of using a high-speed blender is that it will blend these in completely. Kale is incredibly nutritious and is a wonderful addition to a green smoothie; it has a stronger flavor, though, and its taste probably will not go unnoticed. Do remember, though, that you should not go overboard with raw greens in your diet. (Review chapter 26 for an explanation of why.) Also remember that you'll assimilate the calcium in the greens better if your smoothie contains some healthy fat.

Something else to consider is the addition of protein to your smoothie. Adding a protein component is optional, but it helps balance your blood sugar and makes your smoothie more of a meal. I personally do not do well with fruit-only smoothies, and always need to add some sort of protein. I am not a big fan of most protein powders—I don't like the way they taste—but they are good for adding protein to smoothies. Stick to those that are made with grass-fed whey (I don't recommend soy protein powder) if you are going to use them.

Another protein option is raw egg yolks, but only from very fresh, local, free-range eggs! Raw egg yolks are high in omega-3s, and the risk of salmonella from trusted sources is very low. Recall from chapter 23, however, that egg whites are best consumed cooked. Other ingredients you can add to increase the protein and healthy fat content of your smoothie are plain organic yogurt, kefir, good quality milk (raw or organic from grass-fed cows), and nuts and seeds (or nut and seed butters or milks).

If you like, you can also add any of the following to your smoothie: organic coconut milk or coconut oil (good sources of healthy fats), coconut flour (a good source of fiber, but don't use too much or your smoothie will be more like a pudding), raw organic cacao powder or cacao nibs, maca powder (thought to be good for improving stamina), goji berry powder (high in antioxidants), ground flaxseeds (good source of fiber and essential fatty acids), local bee pollen (can help to strengthen your immunity), spirulina or other greens powders (cleansing and nourishing), and aromatics, including fresh mint, ground cinnamon, and fresh or ground ginger. Raw organic oats can also be blended into a smoothie if you eat grains—this increases the fiber content, and oats contain B vitamins, which help combat stress.

Adding a sweetener to your smoothie is probably not necessary, but a small amount of raw honey or maple syrup may be added if you like. You could also use some soaked dried dates or figs to sweeten your smoothie naturally; ripe avocado adds a little sweetness and is a way to give smoothies a naturally creamy consistency, as well.

QUICK REVIEW

⇥ There's a lot that can go wrong with a smoothie. Many are extremely high in carbohydrates and are not a good replacement for a meal or snack. Instead, make smoothies with fruit, a wholesome form of protein, and some healthy fat, plus your choice of nutrient-dense additions.

⇥ Greens are good in smoothies, too (but remember you don't want to eat the same greens all the time, and you don't want to eat *all* your greens raw).

CHOCOLATE-RASPBERRY SMOOTHIE

Serves 1 or 2

I enjoy this smoothie when it's made with my Homemade Yogurt (page 39), but you can experiment with raw milk, kefir, nut milk, or coconut milk for all or part of the liquid, as well. Turn this into a green smoothie by adding a handful or two of any greens you like. Whatever you do, don't skip the raw cacao powder. I can't say enough good things about it—it's high in magnesium, iron, fiber, and antioxidants. Another bonus: As Tyler Graham and Drew Ramsey noted in their book The Happiness Diet, *when raspberries are paired with chocolate, the antioxidants in both are even more effective.*

1 cup/240 ml plain yogurt, *store-bought or homemade (page 39), or kefir, nut milk, or raw or pasteurized whole milk*

1 banana, *preferably fair trade*

1 cup fresh or frozen raspberries

1 yolk of a farm-fresh free-range egg *(optional)*

1 to 2 tbsp raw cacao powder

Ice or water *(optional)*

1 In a blender, blend the yogurt, banana, raspberries, egg yolk, and cacao powder well, adding ice or water to produce the desired consistency.

33 / DEAL WITH THE DAIRY DILEMMA

WE ARE CERTAINLY BOMBARDED WITH MIXED MESSAGES when it comes to dairy, aren't we? We've got our favorite celebrities (with their adorable white mustaches) asking us over and over if we've "got milk?" And we're told that dairy products must be consumed if we're to have strong bones. But we've also been told that the saturated fat in dairy is bad, so many of us dutifully purchase and eat dairy products that are fat free.

At the same time, we've also got a number of health "gurus" telling us that if we want to be healthy, we shouldn't be consuming dairy products at all. They say our bodies are not designed to drink cow's milk. They point out that a great many people lack the enzyme lactase, and are therefore lactose intolerant, and that milk proteins are highly allergenic. They also argue that commercial milk can't possibly be good for us, since it contains hormones, antibiotics, herbicides, and pesticides (because of the unnatural ways dairy cows are medicated and fed). They believe milk makes the body acidic and is therefore actually bad for our bones. They offer up numerous—supposedly superior—alternatives to dairy for getting calcium into the body.

Then there's yet another group of folks who believe that dairy is indeed extremely nutritious, but that we shouldn't be drinking modern industrial milk. Instead, we should seek out milk and milk products from cows that are raised humanely without the administration of antibiotics and hormones, and who are also grazed on pasture. This means buying milk that's organic and grass fed, or possibly even going one step further and sourcing grass-fed, organic milk that's also raw (in other words, unpasteurized and unhomogenized).

After reading a number of thorough and quite excellent accounts of the history of milk, I must say that I agree with the third group. I think milk can be an extremely healthy food, but the type of milk and dairy products we choose to consume is of the utmost importance. I first tried raw milk about ten years ago, but didn't have a way to get it on a regular basis. Since learning of a local source a few years ago, I've been drinking it almost exclusively.

I understand that many people think drinking milk that hasn't been pasteurized is a bad—dangerous, even—idea, but keep in mind that when milk is heated to kill off potentially harmful bacteria, beneficial bacteria are also destroyed. Pasteurization kills enzymes, as well, including those that help with the digestion of dairy. (I've heard many reports of people with a lactose intolerance being able to drink raw milk without a problem.) Raw milk is also said to boost the immune system, and it appears to be tolerated by many who have allergies or sensitivities to commercial milk, though it's hard to pinpoint exactly why this is the case.

Proponents of raw milk claim that it's way more nutritious than its pasteurized and homogenized counterpart, but I must admit that I found it very hard to get solid, third-party verified information about the nutrient content of raw versus regular milk while I was researching this book. To the best of my knowledge, they do contain the same amount of calcium and protein.

I'm not going to discuss all the additional potential benefits of drinking raw milk here because you can find that information elsewhere, but I will say that I drink my milk raw because I personally believe it's a safe and healthy food and I enjoy the way it tastes. In addition, I want to support the farmers in my community who take great care of their cows (the cows in commercial dairies are often kept in truly deplorable conditions) and who do what it takes to make clean raw milk available to me. This is not to say that *you* should drink raw milk. Please do your own research to determine if it's the right choice for you.

If you can't find or don't want to drink raw milk, I suggest purchasing organic milk from pastured cows that's been either pasteurized and homogenized, or only pasteurized. Buying organic milk from pastured cows will ensure that it's free of antibiotics and hormones, and that the cows eat a diet primarily of grass (instead of the corn, soy, and many other undesirable things that commercial dairy cows are fed). The milk fat of cows that graze on grass is high in a number of nutrients, including beneficial omega-3 fatty acids and conjugated linolenic acid (CLA, which has been shown to fight cancer, promote muscle growth, and reduce abdominal body fat). Organic butter from pastured cows is a particularly good source of these nutrients. The milk fat of cows that eat corn and soybeans does not have a healthy fatty acid profile.

Some people avoid homogenized milk because it's potentially more allergenic and because it's been implicated as a causal factor in heart disease. Studies have, indeed, found that drinking raw milk is inversely correlated with allergic reactions and asthma, but I could not find any that support the theory that homogenization is linked to atherosclerosis.

As I have stated elsewhere in this book, I believe that if you eat dairy, you should always consume it full fat. I know this flies in the face of what many nutritionists recommend, but I feel strongly that the fat that's naturally present in high quality milk is not unhealthy. If you opt for commercially available organic milk, then buy whole milk (not reduced fat and definitely not skim), because the fat is where many of the nutrients are (including the omega-3s and CLA). If you decide to drink raw milk, you'll find that the cream floats to the top of the milk, and you just need to give it a few good shakes to disperse the fat throughout.

I drank skim milk at one point in my life, but I cannot imagine doing so now because I think it tastes terrible. Contrary to what we've heard in the mainstream media for a long time, low-fat versions of traditional foods do not support health; a diet full of them is not only unsatisfying but also typically upsets blood sugar and insulin levels. This ultimately makes it hard, if not impossible, to maintain a healthy weight (and it also leads to other health issues).

It's important to note that historically, milk was not consumed fresh in many parts of the world. It was (and continues to be) transformed into yogurt and other cultured dairy foods, as well as cheeses. The cream on top was cultured and enjoyed with other foods or churned into butter (the buttermilk that remained was drunk or utilized in recipes). There's much wisdom in this; these derivatives of milk have always been prized for their abilities to nourish the body, and they are generally well tolerated, even by those who don't digest milk very well on its own. To reiterate the point about choosing whole dairy foods: Think about how many hundreds if not thousands of years our ancestors around the world have been enjoying full-fat dairy products. Low-fat dairy has been available for only a short time (since the last century). It's not a natural food.

Recall from chapter 11 that dairy is one of the most common food sensitivities. Be aware that many people who have problems with gluten find themselves in trouble with dairy, too, because their digestive system is already compromised. I mention this just so you can keep in mind that even if you go out of your way to buy the healthiest dairy products, they still might not work for you.

→ There's no reason to deprive yourself of dairy if you are not allergic, intolerant, or sensitive to it and you enjoy it.

→ Be sure to choose full-fat organic dairy foods, preferably from pastured cows.

→ Raw milk is another option; do some research so you can determine if it might be right for you.

DO-IT-YOURSELF CRÈME FRAÎCHE

Makes 2 cups/480 ml

True crème fraîche is a type of cultured cream that originated in France, where raw cream was allowed to ferment and thicken with the help of naturally occurring bacteria. This isn't something most people can successfully do at home, but a great crème fraîche stand-in (I call it DIY crème fraîche) can be made at home with store-bought cream and buttermilk. You can also use yogurt instead of buttermilk as the culture. A few tablespoons of a previous batch of DIY crème fraîche will work, too. Whichever way you make it, be sure to use a good quality cultured dairy product as your starter, or your cream won't thicken well and will lack the characteristic tang of crème fraîche. For this reason, use cultured buttermilk, and not a buttermilk that is the by-product of butter, which isn't cultured.

I use this crème fraîche all the time in my kitchen: I swirl it into soups (such as the Silky Carrot Soup on page 149) and sauces (it does not curdle when boiled due to its high fat content). I add it to Mexican dishes in lieu of sour cream, and dollop it on desserts instead of whipped cream. It's also good in egg dishes (such as Smoked Wild Salmon and Crème Fraîche Omelet, page 83).

2 cups/480 ml cream, *preferably raw, or at least organic and not ultrapasteurized*

1 tbsp cultured buttermilk

EQUIPMENT

One 1-pt/480-ml glass canning jar with a screw-top lid, metal or BPA-free plastic

1 Clean the glass jar and lid in hot, soapy water, or use the hottest setting on your dishwasher.

2 Pour the cream into the glass jar and stir in the buttermilk. Cover the jar and allow it to sit while the cultures go to work and thicken the cream. If your kitchen is warm, it may take only 12 hours for this to happen. If the ambient temperature is cool, however, it may take 1 or 2 days, or even a little more. It has taken up to 2½ days in my kitchen. Remove the lid and check the progress of the culture every 6 hours or so after the initial 12 hours. On occasion I have left it a bit too long, and a slight off odor was apparent when the cream thickened. If this happens, just scoop off and discard the very top layer. (Some recipes call for heating the cream before you add the buttermilk, which is said to enhance the culturing, but I don't do this because I like to use raw cream.)

34 / SCRATCH THE SODA

MANY PEOPLE—even seemingly health-conscious people—drink soda every day. It doesn't really matter if you drink regular or diet sodas; *I want you to quit.*

There are so many things I don't like about soda. At the top of the list: There are more than 3 tbsp of sugar in a 12-oz/360-ml soda. You already know about the many ways in which sugar can mess up your body, so why gulp down a beverage that contains such a crazy amount (and who even stops at 12 oz/360 ml)? To make matters worse, the sugar in soda is not even pure sugar; it's high-fructose corn syrup (HFCS), and HFCS is reputed to affect the metabolism even more adversely than sugar. Another problem with soft drinks is that people who drink them tend to do so in lieu of drinking water and other beverages that are health-promoting; this can easily lead to dehydration.

Back in my dieting days, I drank lots of diet soda. I gave it up long ago, though, and I definitely think you should, too. As I mentioned in chapter 14, artificial sweeteners like aspartame are made from chemicals that are potentially toxic to your brain and nervous system. Artificial sweeteners are also incredibly addictive (which explains why so many folks are hooked on the diet soda habit). But I think the real shame is that using sugar substitutes doesn't even aid weight loss (or prevent weight gain). There are many reasons for this; one of them seems to be that tasting something sweet—whether from sugar or an artificial sweetener—enhances the appetite. Artificial sweeteners also do nothing to address—and may even worsen—sugar cravings and dependence. I far prefer to use natural sweeteners.

Both regular and diet soft drinks contain artificial colors, and they're also high in acids that are bad for your bones (calcium is pulled out of your bones to buffer the acid, and over time this weakens them and contributes to osteoporosis). Acidic beverages like soda also have the potential to erode your tooth enamel. Studies have shown that the combination of carbonation and caffeine in cola-type drinks is particularly problematic for bone health.

There are so many other things you can drink—some of which are also bubbly and sweet—that are not nearly as bad for you as commercial soda. There are many high quality natural sodas on the market.

In my home, we rely on sparkling water mixed with organic juice when we're looking for something like a soda. I generally mix 3 parts sparkling water, which we make in a SodaStream, with 1 part juice. I also make homemade syrups from natural sweeteners, fruits, and herbs, and we stir these into sparkling water, too. I do allow my kids to have a soda once in a while when we're out to dinner, but I never keep it in the house.

If you drink regular or diet soda for the caffeine, then I suggest you do some thinking about what's going on to make you need it, and look for alternative ways to boost your energy. Make sure to get regular exercise, sleep more, eat well, and manage your stress (review chapter 5 for a refresher on the connection between stress and fatigue). Always remember that water should be your beverage of choice (go back and read chapter 3 if you need to review why).

A 2012 study in the British medical journal The Lancet *found that in the United States, per capita consumption of soft drinks has increased by about 400 percent in the last fifty years. Soda is inextricably linked to our obesity epidemic and to many of our other health woes (such as cancer, diabetes, and cardiovascular disease).*

It's important to know that all carbonated beverages—even seltzer water—are acidic. My feeling is that for most people, it is fine to drink seltzer in moderation, but make sure to drink still (noncarbonated) water, too. If you know you have low bone density, however, avoid all carbonated drinks and focus on building bone density via a nutrient-dense diet and an exercise program that highlights strength training.

QUICK REVIEW

↪ Soda is full of high-fructose corn syrup (or potentially unsafe artificial sweeteners) as well as chemicals and acids that are bad for your bones.

↪ If you drink soda on a regular basis, I want you to quit.

↪ Water is a much better bet for hydration.

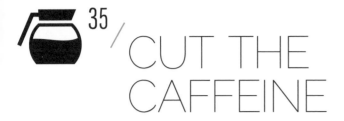

35 / CUT THE CAFFEINE

RIGHT ABOUT NOW YOU ARE THINKING THAT YOU HATE ME. I took away your wheat, your white sugar, and most recently, your diet soda. In your mind you are pleading, "Please don't take my coffee!" Well, you don't have to worry. I am not going to take it away. I *am* going to ask you to evaluate your consumption, however, and see if you can cut back.

Coffee is not inherently bad. In fact, it has some true health benefits because it's a potent antioxidant. A Finnish study linked coffee consumption to a decreased risk of dementia; other studies have shown that coffee drinking is inversely proportional to the development of diabetes and heart disease. Caffeinated black and green tea also have antioxidant properties (green tea more than black), and I enjoy both of them on a daily basis.

Here's the thing, though: The caffeine in coffee (and tea to a lesser extent) is also a stimulant, and many people abuse it. Instead of getting more sleep or dealing appropriately with their stressors, they reach for cup after cup of coffee. Too much caffeine can raise your blood pressure and blood sugar; it can also cause anxiety, irritability, and a number of other health problems.

You already know how I feel about caffeinated sodas; they spell trouble for your health, so you should not drink them. But when it comes to coffee and tea, I think you just need to work on moderation and on choosing healthful varieties. Know that too much caffeine can negatively affect your sleep and your adrenal glands (recall that your adrenal glands are generally overworked, since they're called on in times of stress to secrete adrenaline and cortisol). When you drink coffee or other caffeinated beverages, this only serves to stimulate them further. You don't want to work your adrenals too hard because if you do, they'll become fatigued and you will get sick. So make sure you don't overdo it when it comes to caffeine.

Another problem with caffeinated drinks is that they can also suppress your appetite. If you drink a lot of coffee in the morning, you might be more likely to skip breakfast and not eat enough real food overall. If that is true for you, back off on the coffee.

If you do want to continue drinking coffee, make sure to choose fair-trade, shade-grown coffee to ensure workers are paid a fair wage for their product, and to show your support for sustainable farming practices. (Coffee is a shrub that naturally prefers the shade, but rainforests have been clear-cut to increase yield in recent years. This has been devastating both to the land and to migratory bird populations.) Also, it is important to drink organic coffee or tea so that you do not ingest unwanted chemicals. But don't go overboard, especially in the afternoon and evening (so the caffeine doesn't affect your sleep). And definitely avoid coffee if you are pregnant or are trying to become pregnant.

A final word: Watch what you put in your coffee and tea. Real milk or cream is much healthier than fake creamers. And use a small amount of unrefined sweetener, if any. I take my tea with raw milk and honey from my bees.

QUICK REVIEW

→ Examine your caffeine intake. Be sure to drink only moderate amounts of caffeinated beverages, if you drink them.

→ Don't rely on caffeine to give you a boost when you're tired or stressed; instead, work on the natural measures that will energize you, such as getting more sleep, proper exercise, and enough exposure to the sun and eating a nourishing diet.

→ Don't drink coffee or tea to the exclusion of water and other healthy hydrating beverages.

36 / GET FRESH AIR EVERY DAY

DO YOU GET FRESH AIR EVERY DAY? Many of us don't; we spend nearly all our time inside. Whether we're at home, at school, at work, or in the car (or on a bus or train getting from point A to point B), if we're not spending any time outside, then we're breathing stagnant air and being exposed to numerous potentially toxic chemicals.

Unless you live in a city that's very polluted, the air outside is fresh. Our bodies need fresh air because it cleanses our lungs. Breathing in fresh air also helps to oxygenate the blood and the brain.

It's important get some fresh air as often as possible, and definitely every day. As long as you make getting some fresh air a high priority, this should not be hard to do. If all you have time to do is stand outside your office building and take a few deep breaths, that's better than nothing. But if you can, go for a stroll. Or hang out with your kids in the yard or in a park. And you eat at least three meals a day, yes? How about having one of them outside (weather permitting, of course)?

If you do live somewhere with poor air quality, make sure to escape to an area with cleaner air as frequently as possible: the countryside, mountains, and beach come to mind. When you are there, spend as much time breathing in the crisp, fresh air as you can. I suggest even sleeping outside, if possible.

If you can use your "fresh air time" to get some exercise in, that's great. How about going for a bike

Recall from chapter 5 that the way you breathe directly affects the pH of your blood. According to natural health expert Annemarie Colbin, you need the proper balance of breathing in and out in order to keep your pH in the optimal range. So when you get fresh air, make sure to focus on breathing deeply on both the in and out breaths.

ride or a hike? If you can't seem to get outside often enough, then at least open the doors and windows of your home whenever possible to increase the ventilation and bring in some fresh air.

Keeping houseplants is a great way to freshen up the air in your home. A study by the National Aeronautics and Space Administration (NASA) and the Associated Landscape Contractors of America found that many common plants are able to remove toxic pollutants, including benzene, carbon monoxide, and formaldehyde, from the air. The recommended plants include English ivy, bamboo and reed palms, Boston ferns, spider plants, weeping figs, and philodendrons. In a home of approximately 2,000 sq ft/186 sq m, you should have ten to fifteen plants (two to three small plants or one large plant per room).

I also highly recommend sleeping with your windows open. This gives your body access to beneficial fresh air during the nighttime hours. Plus, many people report they sleep better when they keep their bedroom on the cool side.

The chemicals used in building materials and furnishings are very poorly regulated and really haven't been adequately tested for safety. Many of these chemicals are proven endocrine disruptors and can upset the delicate balance of hormones in the body. For this reason, it's really important to keep your home well ventilated.

QUICK REVIEW

→ Go outside every day and get some fresh air.

→ Don't skip this one just because it's winter—bundle up so you can still get outside. Open the windows to bring some fresh air into your home (and give sleeping with your windows open a try); keeping houseplants is helpful, too.

→ When you're out in the fresh air, take long, slow, deep breaths in and out. This brings the maximum amount of oxygen into your body and helps maintain a healthy, balanced pH in your blood.

37 / CONNECT WITH
NATURE

CONNECTING WITH NATURE IS SECOND NATURE TO MANY OF US. We crave time outside because it's calming and brings us joy. I wasn't always a "nature person;" I grew up in New York City and really did not fall in love with spending time outdoors until I went away to college. I fell hard and fast then, and it's been difficult for me to live in a city ever since.

I currently reside in a small Hudson Valley town in New York, surrounded by a few acres on which I keep flower and vegetable gardens, chickens, and a honeybee hive. Very close by are wonderful hiking trails, swimming holes, and amazing places to go rock climbing. Connecting with nature on a regular basis is extremely important to me, and this is why I've chosen to live where I do.

I don't need scientific studies to confirm the fact that being in nature contributes to happiness, but they do exist; time in nature has also been shown to help alleviate stress and improve memory. Sadly, I don't think most people connect with nature nearly enough these days; it's just so easy to spend time indoors tethered to various forms of technology.

It's really important to disconnect from all those amenities of modern life every now and then and get outdoors, though. For one thing, getting out in nature will help you get your daily allotment of fresh air. It will also make it more likely that you'll be exposed to the sun (and you know how important this is thanks to chapter 7).

If you have kids, bring them with you when you go outside; children can benefit tremendously from connecting with nature. Playing outside helps to combat obesity in kids and appears to improve the focus of children dealing with attention-related issues. It's great to bring kids along on trips to farms (who doesn't love to go apple or pumpkin picking in the fall?) so they can connect to where their food comes from. And one more thing: Fostering a lifelong love of the outdoors in our children is desirable because kids who are more connected with nature will be more likely to appreciate and help protect our planet when they grow up.

Whenever I am feeling stressed or tired, or when I am having a hard time getting stuff done, I go outside. I find that being in nature energizes and reinvigorates me. Keep in mind that you don't actually have to be outside to connect with nature, though. Sure, you can't get fresh air or vitamin D if you're not outside, but you can benefit from simply having a view of something natural. Studies show that classrooms and offices with a view of a park or even a single tree foster a better environment for learning and working.

Going barefoot outdoors can be beneficial to your health. Studies show that most shoes aren't actually good for your feet. (Apparently, just about all shoes cause you to alter your natural gait. High heels and flip-flops are probably the worst; people who wear these types of shoes a lot are more prone to pain in the foot and ankle.) Walking barefoot in nature can be great for your mind as well as your body; think about how amazing it feels to be barefoot in the sand. If you are not comfortable going barefoot outside, consider wearing shoes that simulate going barefoot.

QUICK REVIEW

- Spend some time in nature on a regular basis.
- Connecting with nature is a great way to decrease stress, elevate your mood, and feel connected with the planet.
- How you connect with nature is up to you; try to go outside to exercise (or just to play), to garden, or to spend time in wild places, as often as you can.

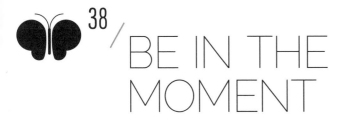

38 / BE IN THE MOMENT

DO YOU KNOW WHAT IT FEELS LIKE to completely lose yourself in a task? To be so fully immersed in doing what you're doing that all your attention is focused on the present? If so, then you know what I am referring to when I say you should spend more time in the moment.

Children are excellent role models for how to be in the moment. If you observe a group of young kids playing, I think you'll agree that there's little chance their minds are elsewhere. They're hyperfocused—they're in the moment! Adults, however, generally stink at just being; it's really hard for us to put our full attention on what's going on right now because we spend most of our time either pining for the past or worrying about the future.

Here's the thing, though: You can't change the past and you can't control the future. All you can do is be . . . here . . . now. There are other terms for being in the moment. Maybe you've heard it referred to as being mindful, or being fully present. Whatever you call it, being in the moment can enhance your health and your life in numerous ways.

If you are stressed, rushed, or upset while you are eating, your digestion can suffer. It's best to eat in a relaxed atmosphere (and definitely not while you are driving). Make sure to sit down during meals. Go ahead and converse with family and friends, but don't forget to focus on your food, too.

What if you were in the moment for every meal, and your focus was on your food and only your food while you ate? Imagine how much you'd enjoy your meal, and how much better it would be digested. You'd pay attention to how your body was feeling with each bite, and you might even eat less as a result. You wouldn't eat on the run or in the car. Think about it: The car is absolutely the worst place to eat because your mind is supposed to be on the road.

And what about each and every other thing you do, aside from eating, at each and every moment of every day? Can you imagine what your life would be like if you did all of it with mindfulness?

Not too long ago, I came face to face with the realization that I have a tendency to overcomplicate my life; I simply try to do too much. When I am so busy rushing through all the tasks I want to get done, I can't enjoy what I'm doing at any given moment. And I can't fully participate in my life.

So I decided to stop saying "yes" to everything, and I strongly suggest you do the same; we're all over-filling our proverbial plates these days. As I mentioned previously, saying "no" more often is a good way to decrease stress. Of course not all stressors are under our control, but many are. Take a good hard look at your to-do lists and see if you can pare them down so that they are actually doable. Then commit yourself to doing all that you do in a fully present manner, without letting your mind wander to other things.

Did you know that humans are not actually meant to multitask? Our brains can't handle doing more than one thing at a time. Multitasking does not make us more efficient; it distracts us and leads to a decrease in productivity. It also makes it impossible to be in the moment.

For me, being in the moment means not turning my thoughts to sweeping the floor when my daughter is telling me about her day, or working on my laptop when I am watching a movie with my husband, or starting a bread-baking project two minutes before I have to head out the door. When it's time to sweep, I sweep, and I give that sweeping all my attention. I've learned that it's possible to find joy in the simplest of tasks if you do them mindfully. Try being mindful when you do dishes or fold laundry, and I think you'll find these chores can be relaxing, not annoying.

QUICK REVIEW

⮕ Practice being mindful during meals so you can fully enjoy your food, digest it better, and maybe even eat less.

⮕ Be mindful when you work, and you'll be able to eliminate the distractions that keep you from getting things done. Be mindful when you're with friends and family, and you'll get more out of your relationships.

⮕ Simplify your life by not multitasking, and by saying "no" more often, so that you can focus on doing one thing at a time and doing it well.

39 / LEAVE A SMALLER FOOTPRINT

I DON'T WANT TO BE OVERLY DRAMATIC, but the Earth is in serious trouble right now. At the time of this writing, severe weather events are happening more and more frequently, and this is evidence that climate change is here. Scientists have been telling us for years that if we do not change the habits that are destroying the planet, there will be no turning back. But we haven't really been listening.

I do believe that we all should—and must—continue to take steps to live in an eco-conscious manner. Our individual actions do make a difference. If I had written this chapter five years ago, I might have taken a fairly lighthearted approach to suggesting ways you can decrease your carbon footprint. While I no longer think being lighthearted is going to cut it, I am still going to share with you some things you can do to help the planet. Nothing here really represents a sacrifice; in fact, lessening your impact on the Earth goes hand in hand with improving the quality of your life.

TIPS FOR REDUCING YOUR CARBON FOOTPRINT

Contemplate your car. If you can let go of your vehicle, this is obviously the best option. If going without a car isn't possible, do your research and decide whether you and the environment would be better off with a different one. Swapping out a car with poor fuel economy for a more efficient option will have a positive impact on the planet as well as on your wallet. If a more fuel-efficient car (new or used) is simply not in the cards, make a commitment to simply driving less (reduced number of car trips = smaller carbon footprint). Use public transportation, walk, bike, or carpool as often as possible.

Bring your own bags. Almost a trillion plastic bags are used worldwide each year. These never break down completely; they pollute our environment and harm our wildlife, so why use them? Bring your own reusable shopping bags to the store instead.

Don't buy bottled water. Plastic bottles are wasteful and may leach toxic chemicals into your water. Drink the free water from your tap (a good filter will remove any bad stuff) in refillable BPA-free water bottles instead. Make it another one of your "green missions" to bring your own mug when you go out for coffee or tea, and just think of all the plastic and paper cups you'll keep out of the garbage.

Carbon dioxide (CO2) is a greenhouse gas that causes heat to be trapped in the Earth's lower atmosphere, contributing to global warming. Your carbon footprint is a measure of how much CO2 is produced to support the way you live. Reducing your carbon footprint means living in a way that has less of a negative impact on the Earth. You can calculate your current carbon footprint at Earthlab's website: www.earthlab.com/createprofile/reg.aspx.

QUICK REVIEW

→ If you are an eco-disaster, it is never too late to change.

→ There are so many habits you can adopt—such as changing your transportation methods, bringing your own bags to the store, and avoiding bottled water—to reduce your carbon footprint.

→ Making these changes will benefit not just the environment but also your health and quite often your wallet, too.

40 / BE ECO-FRIENDLY AT HOME

WE ALL WANT TO LIVE IN A COMFORTABLE HOME—a place where we can enjoy spending our free time (and for those of use who work at home, our work time, too). While many folks feel their habits at home do not affect the planet, this really could not be further from the truth. There are many ways to be eco-friendly at home, and every little change you make will matter.

Strive to make your home energy efficient; this will help to reduce greenhouse gases and conserve the planet's resources (it will also save you money). Improve the insulation in your home, so that when it's chilly, heat isn't lost through your walls and roof. Turn lights off when you leave a room. Use energy-efficient appliances and lightbulbs. Unplug electronics when not in use. Don't run your dishwasher or do the laundry unless you have a full load. Use a clothesline to dry clothes instead of using the dryer whenever possible. Have your furnace serviced annually to ensure it's running properly. Don't automatically crank up the thermostat when you're cold; try putting on a sweater instead.

Next, cut down on the waste you produce. You know the saying, "Reduce, reuse, and recycle"? Well, it's time to put these words into daily practice. Put a stop to your junk mail. Buy in bulk when possible to cut down on packaging. Learn how to compost (more on this in chapter 44). Eliminate the use of items such as paper towels (replace these with dish towels you can toss in the laundry). Use cloth napkins instead of paper ones. If you are having company and you just don't want to wash a lot of dishes, look for single-use plates that are biodegradable and can be added to your compost.

Don't use cleaning agents made with toxic chemicals that are dangerous to both the environment and your health. Purchase those made from naturally derived ingredients or make your own. I talk more about this in chapter 45.

Reconsider your carpets. Most are manufactured with volatile organic compounds (VOCs)—chemicals that can be detected in trace amounts in the air for years to come. This fact, combined with the reality that carpets trap dirt and allergens, might encourage you to avoid carpeting altogether. At the very least, look for carpeting that is environmentally friendly—made from either recycled materials or wool, and anchored with low-VOC adhesive. Low-VOC carpet "tiles" are another good option.

When painting, choose nontoxic paints. More and more companies are offering non- or low-VOC alternatives. These typically require fewer coats and have minimal odor compared to paints of the past. All-natural milk paints (paints made from the milk protein casein) are another good chemical-free choice.

Keeping lots of houseplants helps to purify the air in your home. Review chapter 36 for more information on how houseplants improve air quality.

Hopefully you are spending more time in the kitchen preparing real food, so you'll want to pay particular attention to cooking in greener ways. Some things to think about: Use your oven less by eating more raw foods, cooking on the stove top, or using a smaller countertop or toaster oven whenever possible. Try to use the oven only when cooking several dishes at once.

Cover your pots with a lid when you are cooking to keep the heat in, and hand wash your dishes, or at least don't run the dishwasher unless it's full. Interestingly enough, the microwave appears to be quite eco-friendly. (I don't cook in mine, but I do use it for heating water for tea, and for occasionally reheating foods stored in glass containers.) Crock-Pots are convenient, and they're pretty energy efficient, as well. When grilling, natural gas or propane are cleaner, greener choices than charcoal.

QUICK REVIEW

⟡ Make sure your home is energy efficient and cut down on the waste you produce.

⟡ Limit environmental toxins by avoiding most cleaning agents, being careful about carpeting, and choosing nontoxic paints.

⟡ In the kitchen, use green cooking techniques such as lidded cooking and batch baking. Eating more of your food raw is another way to be green in the kitchen.

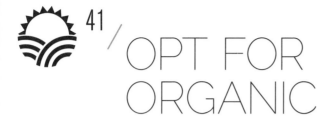

41 / OPT FOR ORGANIC

I GROW MY OWN ORGANIC VEGETABLES; keep my own pastured, organically fed chickens and my own bees; and buy additional organic produce because it is free of toxins. I don't want to ingest pesticides when I eat, and I don't want my kids to, either. I also buy organic dairy and meat to avoid toxins from pesticides (which concentrate in fats), and because the quality of the fats is higher (there are more omega-3s, for example) and organic dairy and meat products contain no antibiotics or hormones. Another reason I buy organic food is to avoid GMOs.

But eating organic is not just about the health of *my* family (or yours)—it's about the health of everyone who's involved in growing and harvesting our foods. It's also about the health of the planet as a whole. And it's about taste! That's why I believe you should eat organic to the extent that you can afford it, as often as possible.

The soil organic produce is grown in is generally higher in nutrients (from practices like enriching it with compost and green "manures," and from crop rotation). But it's unclear whether produce grown organically is more nutritious than conventional.

That shouldn't stop you from buying organic, though. The question of whether or not organic foods contain more vitamins and minerals should only play a small part in your decision to eat organic. As I stated above, it's very important to eat organic animal foods and fats in order to avoid toxins. I also think it's crucial to buy organic versions of the produce items on the Environmental Working Group's "Dirty Dozen" list (which has actually been expanded to include fourteen foods, and can be found here: www.ewg.org/foodnews/summary.php).

It's important to keep in mind, however, that locally grown, conventional produce may sometimes be a better choice than organic produce. Even though apples are on the "Dirty Dozen" list, I'll take apples from local farms over organic ones flown in from who knows where any day (but I look for apples that are low spray, and I always make sure to clean them with a produce wash designed to remove any pesticide residue). Also, some farms don't have an organic certification for whatever reason (including the expense of pursuing one), but the foods they sell are of the highest quality.

Every time you eat, you have the opportunity to invest in your health. *So you should eat the healthiest foods you can find and afford.* I believe the healthiest foods are going to be organic foods that you grow yourself, or that you purchase from a local farm or farmers' market. If procuring food this way isn't possible, then the supermarket is a fine place to shop, as long as you buy real food. Eating real food is so important, even if it's not organic.

QUICK REVIEW

⇢ Opt for organic as often as possible. Grow your own organic food, if you can, and shop organic farms and farmers' markets.

⇢ It is particularly important to choose organic when you buy fats, oils, and animal foods including dairy and meat.

⇢ Make sure you also buy organic when shopping for the fruit and vegetables on the Environmental Working Group's "Dirty Dozen" list.

42 / GET CLOSER TO YOUR FOOD

I'VE NEVER CLAIMED TO BE A LOCAVORE: I eat many foods that are not local, especially during the cold months of the year. But to the degree that I am able, I embrace the idea of getting closer to my food by supporting food producers in my community and growing as much of my own food as I can.

Why is it important to get closer to your food? There are a number of reasons: If you choose to eat foods that are locally grown, you'll avoid excess packaging and preservatives. If foods don't need to be transported long distances, less energy (for refrigeration) and less fuel will be expended in getting them to you, which is better for the environment. Eating local bonds you to your community, and local foods usually taste best. While I don't have the stats to prove it, I am also pretty sure that foods picked and enjoyed when they are ripe are more nutritious than those that travel thousands of miles before they're placed on supermarket shelves.

Getting closer to your food means learning about what grows in your area, and when, so that you can eat foods that come from close by when they are in season. How do you do this? You can plant a garden, forage for wild foods, shop farmers' markets, or visit and purchase items right on the farms themselves. Another option is to join a CSA (Community Supported Agriculture) farm. By doing so, you are purchasing a "share" in a farm. You can find more information about CSAs, and locate one in your area, at the Local Harvest website: www.localharvest.org/csa.

If you live in a place with a warm year-round climate, you have a bit of an advantage over those of us who don't. But there are ways to continue to eat locally year-round, even if you live somewhere that is cold in winter. You can learn techniques for winter gardening and for preserving food.

Getting closer to your food does not mean you have to give up eating everything that's not local, though. This just isn't practical for most people. Chocolate, coffee, tea, and spices are examples of foods that you probably would not want to go without, but which certainly are not local for many of us. So when it comes to these foods, buy them, but look for fair-trade and other sustainable options whenever possible. Keep in mind that these aren't very perishable, and they are relatively light, so their transportation doesn't result in as big a carbon foot-print as is the case with some other foods.

While I try not to be a food snob, I just don't think you can compare the taste of tomatoes bought in the supermarket in December to ones you buy from the farmers' market at the height of the summer (and don't even get me started on strawberries). Do I still buy the occasional tomato in December? Yes, I buy the hothouse-grown ones when I am desperate. But generally, I try to wait until my own tomatoes are ready, and then I pretty much gorge myself all season. Do I buy imported foods like pineapples and mangoes? Yes, I do; I love these fruits and would not want to go without them permanently, but I don't buy them often.

I have a long-standing interest in herbal medicine and edible wild plants, so foraging is something I really love to do. I forage because it's fun and a great way to get out and connect with nature. Also, foraged foods are generally very high in nutrients—and they're free. A word of caution, though: There are a lot of poisonous plants out there, and many of them look like their nontoxic counterparts. So buy some guidebooks, or forage with a knowledgeable person until you are really comfortable with what you're doing. Some of my favorite wild plants—ones I think everyone should know how to identify—are pretty common, and extremely nutritious. These include stinging nettle, purslane, violets, chickweed, dandelion greens, day-lily tubers, lamb's-quarters, and clover (both red and white).

I think that the very best way to get closer to your food is to grow some-thing—anything. I know that not everyone has space to garden, but maybe you could have a plot in a community garden, or consider growing some herbs inside or on a balcony.

QUICK REVIEW

⇥ Get closer to your food by choosing locally grown, season-ally available items whenever possible.

⇥ When you eat local, you are benefiting the environment; local foods require less packaging and transportation.

⇥ Gardening and foraging are great ways to get closer to your food; I am a big fan of both.

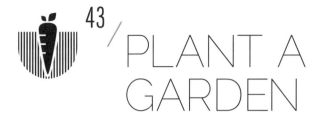

43 / PLANT A GARDEN

I AM NO GARDENING EXPERT, BUT I'VE LEARNED A LOT since my first effort, which consisted of one tomato plant in a container on the deck of a rental home. I'd love to inspire those of you who do have space for a garden to take the plunge. Maybe you're interested, but just don't know where to begin.

Now I know what you're thinking. You are thinking that starting (and maintaining) a garden is *not* simple. And you're not wrong; a garden can be a lot of work. That said, I am really passionate about organic gardening, and I honestly believe this pursuit can change your life. I also believe that once you've built your infrastructure, gardening *can* be simple!

Now I'd be thrilled if you wanted to embark on building a huge garden after reading this chapter, but my goal here is really just to encourage you to grow something—maybe some herbs. Because after you do that, after you get your feet wet, you might be inspired to expand your horizons and grow more. This is what happened to me; it's been about fifteen years since I grew my first tomatoes. Now I have a really big fenced garden with ten raised beds, which are packed with fruits and vegetables!

An organic home garden enhances the look and feel of your home, and an organic vegetable garden feeds your family the healthiest possible produce. Organic gardens also encourage diverse ecosystems, which is great for the environment. A garden can be a small or a large commitment, or something in between. In my experience, however, setting up the garden involves the most work; once that part is done, I don't find gardening to be particularly time-consuming (or maybe it is, but I love it so much that I don't notice!).

I do most of my gardening work on the weekends in the spring and summer. Planting seeds and starter plants takes some time, but other than that,

I spend about ten to fifteen minutes per day mostly trying to stay on top of weeds. Damn those weeds! You can't beat them, so you may as well identify the edible ones and eat them. I mulch the areas around my raised beds very heavily, which cuts down on the weeds a lot.

If you have never gardened before, you might want to start out by gardening in containers, like I did. Or you could start with just one or two raised beds. If you're sure want a bigger garden, spend some time evaluating your property to determine the best site. Planning a successful and beautiful kitchen garden takes time, so don't rush. Look at books or magazines for inspiration, then draw a map of what you'd like your garden to look like, and ask yourself the following questions:

I am intrigued by permaculture, an ecological design system that offers solutions for some of the modern world's most pressing social and environmental issues, including energy conservation, water conservation, and sustainable local food production. Permaculture in the garden involves working with nature, rather than against it, by using techniques such as directly harvesting rainwater and mulching plants heavily with organic materials. Permaculture techniques can be used to create low-maintenance edible gardens that mimic natural ecosystems.

How much sun does your proposed garden site receive? Keep in mind that if it's less than six to eight hours a day, it's probably not an appropriate site for growing vegetables.

What do you want to grow—a few basic veggies or a large assortment of heirloom varieties? I am of the opinion that it's more fun to grow things you can't find in the supermarket. That's why I grow sorrel and lemongrass, for example.

What is your soil like? Getting your soil tested is always a good idea; it's important to know what you are working with in terms of texture, acidity, and the presence of minerals. But you should add nutrients to your soil regardless of the results. In fact, if you take away just one tip from this chapter, let it be that cultivating high-quality soil is the most important thing you can do in your home garden. You don't want to plant in plain old topsoil; you want to mix in lots and lots of compost and other organic matter, such as peat moss or manure. I compost everything I can and love being able to add my compost—and all the wonderful worms that come with it—to my garden beds. The bedding from my chicken coop (the poop mixed in with all the cedar shavings) gets added to my compost every now and then, as well; this is also excellent for the garden.

Are you going to use raised beds? How many will you need? What dimensions will they be? What material will they be made from? I believe raised-bed gardening has many advantages over planting directly in the ground. You'll have greater control over your growing medium—you can fill your beds with high quality topsoil, plus all the organic matter I mentioned earlier. You'll also have better drainage—excess moisture drains more easily from raised beds, which is better for most vegetables and flowers. In raised beds, the soil warms faster, giving you a longer growing season, which is especially important for heat-loving plants like tomatoes (though you may need to cool raised beds down in the heat of summer with mulch). Lastly, raised-bed gardening is easier on the body; you don't need to stoop so much, since the plants are closer to you.

Raised beds should be rectangular. A good width is 4 ft/1.2 m, as it allows you to reach across the bed from either side (you don't want to have to walk in your raised bed, which compacts the soil). If you plan to grow a vining vegetable on a trellis against one of the long sides of the bed, you should probably make your bed narrower. Brett L. Markham, the author of *Mini Farming for Self Sufficiency* (2006), suggests 3½ ft/1 m, so you'll be able to access the trellis.

You can make your beds as high as you like—a higher level is desirable for less mobile individuals or those with back trouble. If you are building more than one raised bed, make sure to leave a pathway wide enough for a wheelbarrow to travel in between your beds.

You can build your own raised beds; there are many materials that work well. Wood such as redwood or cedar is an attractive choice, but keep in mind that wood may rot. Pressure-treated wood lasts longer than untreated wood, but it does contain chemicals that some people find objectionable (it used to contain arsenic, but fortunately, it no longer does). You can paint or stain the wood, but make sure that whatever you use won't contaminate your plants.

Concrete blocks are not as pretty as wood, but they are very durable (and cheap!). You can change the shape of your beds if you use concrete blocks, but they are heavy and you'll need quite a few, which is a disadvantage. Stones make beautiful raised beds, but they, too, are heavy and they can be expensive. Bamboo is an option, and recycled plastic is a very long-lasting and relatively inexpensive option.

You can also make a raised bed without using any material to enclose it, but the shape won't hold as well, and it will be prone to erosion. A good option, if you prefer not to enclose your bed, is to make a raised bed using the sheet-mulching method. Layers of recycled materials, such as newspaper or cardboard, are added to the garden bed to get rid of grass and weeds. The process, also known as lasagna gardening and no-till gardening, also allows you to easily add nutrients to the soil, and it attracts helpful critters such as worms. You can sheet mulch in a raised bed enclosure as well—you'll end up with wonderfully productive soil.

Will you be bringing in soil and compost to fill the beds? How much will you need? If you come to my house on any given day in the spring, you are likely to see a big pile at the end of my driveway. This might be screened topsoil, composted manure, or a mixture of the two. I suggest staying away from buying any of this stuff in bags. It costs much more, and then you have to throw away the plastic bags. You're better off getting it delivered in bulk from a local garden center (if you have access to a pickup truck, you'll save on the delivery fee). You'll be able to estimate how much of everything you need if you give the dimensions of your gardening beds to the person you're ordering the materials from. By the way, wheelbarrowing or shoveling the materials from your piles to your raised beds is a great workout.

How will you water? Can you utilize rain barrels or an irrigation system? I recommend both! You can always use sprinklers, but I find it a bit hard to direct the water exactly where it needs to go. Keep in mind that watering a garden by hand can eat up a lot of time.

Do you have critters that you want to keep out of your garden? Are they small or large? If you need a fence, how high does it need to be, and what will you construct it with? Building a fence to surround our garden was no small task, but it was essential. I have big dogs who enjoy digging, and I did not want them getting into my garden. There is also a huge deer population in our area. Our fence is made of heavy-duty chicken wire, which we buried several inches/centimetres by digging a trench around the perimeter of the garden. We put small stones into the trench on both sides of the fence; this has been very effective in keeping any animals from crawling under it.

As far as smaller garden pests go, I haven't really noticed many problems with "bad bugs" (except when I attempted to grow eggplants). This is possibly due to the fact that I plant marigolds all throughout my vegetable beds (these are said to repel a variety of pests). I also have a perennial flower bed in the center of my garden, and I plant many edible flowers and herbs throughout my vegetable beds: These all seem to attract beneficial insects, and they keep away pests, as well.

How will you maximize space in your new garden? Can you utilize structures that will allow your vegetables to grow vertically—such as cages for tomatoes, cucumbers, and peppers; and fences or trellises for climbing beans and for peas? This is especially important if you don't have a lot of room, but even if you do, it's just good practice to allow veggies to grow up, instead of letting them spread out on the ground, whenever possible.

How much time are you willing to put into the maintenance of your garden? Be realistic and try not to bite off more that you can chew. (If you don't want to spend any time maintaining your own garden, then you can think of your local farmers' market as your garden instead!) If you find that something you need to do is out of your skill set (such as building raised beds or a fence), you can always hire help. Or, if you have like-minded friends, you could organize garden work days on which you help each other with different projects. I have participated in several garden-building days at my children's schools, and it always amazes me how much lighter the work is and how much gets done when there are lots of people on hand to help.

Connecting with other gardeners in your community can be a great way to sort out any questions you have about getting started. I have found that seasoned gardeners love sharing their knowledge and experiences.

QUICK REVIEW

⇨ Grow something! Plant herbs (they are very low maintenance), or try gardening in containers if you're not sure you have a green thumb.

⇨ If you're up for building a garden, my tips can help you get started.

⇨ After you set up your garden, you just need to spend your time planting and harvesting—and controlling the weeds. I recommend eating the weeds over trying to beat them.

SILKY CARROT SOUP

Serves 5 or 6

I love making this creamy carrot soup in the fall, when I begin to crave warm comfort foods. It's just terrific made with freshly harvested carrots from the garden, but if you don't have homegrown carrots, you can certainly use store-bought organic carrots instead.

Carrots are a great source of carotenes, which help to prevent cancer. According to herbalist Susun Weed, they are much more useful to the body when the carrots are cooked, not raw. Carrots also contain some minerals, including boron and calcium. Don't be put off by the crème fraîche or coconut milk. Besides adding a satisfying richness to the soup, these are good quality sources of fat and are essential for helping your body absorb fat-soluble nutrients.

1 tbsp butter, *preferably from pastured cows*

1 tbsp olive oil

1 large onion, *chopped*

2 garlic cloves, *chopped*

1 pound/455 g carrots, *peeled and chopped*

1 large sweet potato, *peeled and chopped (or use an equivalent amount of chopped parsnip or cubed winter squash)*

½ cup/120 ml dry white wine *(such as Chardonnay or Sauvignon Blanc)*

6 cups/1.4 L homemade chicken, turkey, or vegetable stock (page 37), or water

½ cup/120 ml crème fraîche, *homemade (page 124) or store-bought, or organic cream, or coconut milk*

Sea salt and freshly ground black pepper

...continued

1 Melt the butter with the oil in a large soup pot over medium-high heat. Add the onion and sauté, stirring frequently, for about 5 minutes. Add the garlic and sauté for 1 minute more.

2 Add the carrots, sweet potato, and wine and bring to a boil. Reduce the heat to low and cook, stirring every now and then, for 5 minutes, or until some of the wine has cooked off. Add the stock and bring to a boil. Skim the surface of the liquid, if necessary, and return the heat to low. Simmer uncovered for 40 minutes, or until the vegetables are very soft. Remove from the heat.

3 Purée the soup in the pot, using an immersion blender, or allow the soup to cool slightly and purée it in batches in a blender or food processor. Return the puréed soup to the pot and add the crème fraîche. Reheat over medium heat until warmed through, adding more stock if necessary to achieve the desired consistency. Add salt and black pepper to taste before serving.

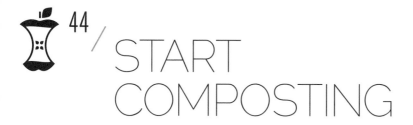

44 / START COMPOSTING

DID YOU KNOW that about one-third of the food that is produced on Earth goes to waste? How sad is that, considering how many people don't have enough to eat in this world? Apparently there are terrible environmental consequences of this waste, as well, since discarded food is a major cause of avoidable carbon dioxide (CO_2) emissions.

While I recognize that composting isn't a solution to the problem, it does keep kitchen and yard wastes out of landfills, plus it's awesome for gardening. I wish more people would compost. It's easy—especially if you've got some outdoor space—so I hope to inspire you to get started with composting if it's not something you already do.

I have been composting for many years, and believe it or not, I am still in awe of the process. I think it's beyond cool that I can take organic matter from my kitchen and yard (plus other surprising places), put it in a pile, and watch it break down into something that I can then add back to my soil to fertilize the plants that have yet to grow. That's recycling at its finest as far as I am concerned.

Composting really is that simple; you are, after all, basically putting things into a pile to rot. But you know what? I don't like describing a compost pile as a mound of rotting waste, because that makes it sound disgusting, and a compost pile isn't disgusting at all.

There are basically two ways to compost: the hot way and the cool way. Cool composting is a slow process (it can take months to a year or more for it to break down). Hot composting speeds things up (your compost is typically finished in one or two months).

My method is more cool than hot. I have a compost pile made from my kitchen scraps, garden and yard clippings, and spent chicken bedding, and I keep adding material to the top of the pile whenever I have it. I keep a plastic container for compost in my kitchen, where I collect all my fruit and veggie discards, eggshells, used tea bags, and coffee grounds. (It's very tightly covered, which is so important, particularly in the summer, as it helps to avoid fruit flies.) I dump these on top of the pile every few days, and turn my pile with a pitchfork whenever I remember (I am trying to be better about this, as it's actually really important to aerate your compost pile). And I water the pile whenever it gets dry. In the winter, I add things to the pile just as in summer, but decomposition obviously slows to a halt when it's very cold.

I like doing things this way because it's easy and free. It doesn't smell bad, and it does not attract unwanted critters (something a lot of people seem to worry about). Remember to never add meat, fish, or any kind of cooked food to your compost, though (if you do, you may indeed see some uninvited "guests").

If you've never composted before, you might get frustrated with how long it takes, and you'll probably be astounded when you see how little compost you actually end up with from what initially seemed like a big pile. But oh, how dark and glorious that compost will be, filled with nutrients and wiggling worms, which are *so* excellent for organic gardening.

If you're not into the idea of having a compost pile because you think they are ugly, you don't have the space, or you're just impatient, you might want to try the hot approach, and buy a bin designed for composting. These are generally made from recycled plastic, and are widely available online and at large gardening centers. In my town, you can also purchase bins at the municipal recycling center. Using a compost bin definitely has some advantages: Turning the contents is easier, so you can do it frequently (yes!). Plus the bin has a lid, so the heat is contained (the hotter things become inside the bin, the sooner you will end up with finished compost that you can use).

If you don't have a garden, and don't see the point of composting, just think of how much less garbage you'll make if you compost the suitable items instead. I am sure you can find a gardening friend who'd be happy to take your compost off your hands, or you could use it to enrich the soil of your potted indoor plants.

City apartment dwellers: You are probably thinking that this info is not for you, but I beg to differ. Look into urban composters designed to be used indoors. Another option is to compost in a worm bin. *Worms Eat My Garbage: How to Set Up and Maintain a Worm Composting System* (2006) by Mary Appelhof is a terrific book.

QUICK REVIEW

⮑ Composting is a great way to recycle instead of throwing away waste, and it's a must if you have an organic garden.

⮑ Composting is very simple and can be done in a pile or a dedicated bin.

⮑ City dwellers can consider urban composters or worm bins.

HOW TO MAKE A SUCCESSFUL COMPOST PILE

Your compost pile should be one-half to two-thirds green, and one-third to one-half brown.

- → The green material (high in nitrogen) can include grass clippings; green plant trimmings; young weeds (best to avoid weeds with seeds); bedding and manure from chickens, cows, and horses; and food scraps, including all raw fruit and veggie scraps, cooked grains, used organic tea bags and leaves, coffee grounds, and eggshells (but *no* meat, bones, dairy products, whole eggs, or oils). Avoid adding large amounts of cooked vegetables or fruit to your compost pile, but a little is just fine.

- → The brown material (high in carbon) can include raked leaves, straw, hay, waste paper and shredded junk mail, wood shavings, newspaper, and cardboard.

For adequate heating, it is best to make a pile about 3 ft/0.9 m square. Water should be added to keep the pile as moist as a wrung-out sponge (use a hose). Keep it covered with a tarp if it's raining a lot and the pile is getting too wet.

When building your pile, layer the greens and browns and add water to help jump-start their breakdown. Then keep an eye on the moisture level and turn the contents with a pitchfork every week or two to make sure it continues to decompose evenly. The more you turn the materials over and get things stirred up, the faster they will decompose.

45 / GREEN YOUR CLEANING

I'VE ALREADY MENTIONED that household cleaning products are a source of potentially harmful chemicals. At best, these may cause acute irritation of the eyes and skin; at worst, long-term exposure to some of these ingredients may contribute to very serious issues, such as reproductive problems and breast cancer, due to their endocrine-disrupting nature. Many cleaning agents also contribute to air and water pollution, and their packaging is not environmentally friendly.

For these reasons, it's important to "green your cleaning," and the best way to do this is to make your own homemade cleaners from common, all-natural ingredients. It's easy and you'll be doing a great thing for the planet. The health of your whole family (including your pets) will benefit, too, and you'll save money.

The main ingredient I use for green cleaning is one I know you already have around: water. It works surprisingly well when combined with a little vegetable oil–based all-purpose liquid soap and elbow grease! The other ingredients I use most often to clean green are baking soda, white vinegar, and salt.

I rarely use more than water for mopping my floors, though sometimes I will add a little vinegar for cleaning the wood. When I need something abrasive (for the sink, oven, and bathtubs, for example), I rely on baking soda. If you mix it with some water into a paste, you have a great alternative to scrubbing products that contain nasty chemicals like hypochlorite (a.k.a. liquid bleach).

Baking soda can also be sprinkled on carpets before vacuuming, and used to whiten laundry. When combined with white vinegar, it can unclog

Many of the products on the market claiming to be nontoxic and eco-friendly contain ingredients with questionable safety records. If you want to check out your favorite store-bought green cleaning agents to see how they rate, visit the website of the Environmental Working Group and search their section on household cleaners (www.ewg .org/guides/cleaners).

drains. I keep large boxes of baking soda on hand because it's so very useful for cleaning (mixed with water, it even makes a substitute for toothpaste).

Vinegar can be mixed with hot water and a bit of liquid soap for cleaning tiles and glass; it also works well for cleaning toilets and will kill mold in the shower or tub. If you don't like the strong scent of vinegar, you can mix it with a few drops of a delectable-smelling natural essential oil (such as lemongrass) in a spritz bottle.

Salt makes a good abrasive (coarse types can be even more effective than baking soda); it works well for cleaning pots and pans. Inexpensive salts are just fine for this purpose—no reason to use more expensive sea salts!

Though I don't own any brass or copper, I have heard that lemon juice makes an excellent polish for these metals.

QUICK REVIEW

⇢ Homemade cleaners help you cut down on the potentially toxic chemicals in your life, and save you money at the same time.

⇢ Try homemade cleaners made from simple ingredients such as water, baking soda, salt, and white vinegar.

⇢ If you prefer to buy your cleaning products, don't assume that a product is eco-friendly or nontoxic just because it claims to be; check the website of the Environmental Working Group to be sure it's safe to use as a household cleaner.

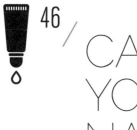

46 / CARE FOR YOUR SKIN NATURALLY

BY NOW YOU WELL KNOW that you shouldn't eat anything that contains ingredients you don't recognize or can't pronounce. Well, the same goes for your skin care products. The scary truth is that just like cleaning products, the vast majority of commercial skin care products contain potentially toxic chemicals, such as phthalate plasticizers and paraben preservatives.

Phthalates are found in eye makeup, nail polish, lotions, and perfume. Parabens are used in thousands of products, including deodorant, shampoo, and hairspray. Both of these are classified as endocrine disruptors. A few other things you should know: Many lipsticks contain lead, hair dye is a suspected carcinogen, and the cotton used in tampons (unless they are organic) is bleached with chlorine.

Most people don't think twice about their personal care products; they assume that if something is on the market, its ingredients have been tested and approved for safety. But this is not the case. On its website, the U.S. Food and Drug Administration (FDA) warns, "*With the exception of color additives and a few prohibited ingredients, a cosmetic manufacturer may use almost any raw material as a cosmetic ingredient and market the product without an approval from the FDA.*"

The skin is the body's largest organ, and it's very thin, so any chemicals in any product that you apply can get into your bloodstream very easily. What's more, many skin care products contain "penetration enhancers," which pretty much guarantee the toxins will find their way to various tissues in the body. As you know, there are a lot of problematic chemicals out in the environment that we can't really do anything about. There might even be chemicals in your home that you can't eliminate. Your skin care products are another story, as are the cleaning products you use and the food you eat. You have 100 percent control over these, so why not choose wisely? This will help you reduce the total number of toxins your body has to deal with on a regular basis.

You would think that the health food store would be a great place to find healthy skin care products—the shelves are packed with various items claiming to be natural and organic, after all—but this isn't necessarily the case. Labels can be misleading. Many of these so-called natural cosmetics contain synthetic ingredients, and even petrochemicals (chemicals derived from petroleum). How do you know if your cosmetics are okay? Check the Environmental Working Group's online safety guide for cosmetics and personal care products. The EWG has reviewed over seven thousand products; search its database at www.ewg.org/skindeep.

In addition to making sure the ingredients in your cosmetics are nontoxic, look for products that don't have synthetic fragrances added. These are very allergenic and their derivatives may be stored in your fatty tissues. Opt for cosmetics in glass containers (not plastic) to limit your exposure to BPA, and don't buy from companies that test their products on animals.

Personal care products that are truly safe can be quite expensive. An alternative is to make your own with high quality, truly natural ingredients. This will save you money, benefit your health, and can be really fun if you like do-it-yourself projects. I've included one of my favorite body scrub recipes on page 160.

Ultimately, it's really important to consider how many personal care products you actually need. I was astounded when I read that a large Environmental Working Group survey found that 25 percent of women use fifteen or more products on their skin *every day*.

MORE TIPS FOR NATURALLY HEALTHY SKIN

Make sure you are drinking enough water and eating lots of fruits and vegetables to keep yourself properly hydrated. Many antioxidants in food help to fight signs of aging: Green tea is a powerful one. It's also important to have plenty of healthy fats in the diet, especially the omega-3s.

I love a hot shower, but heat really dries out your skin and hair. Try showering in tepid or even cold water. If you can't stand being in a cold shower for very long, at least try to make the end of your shower cold.

Organic coconut oil is more than a healthy cooking oil; it is wonderful for the skin! I use a small amount on my face as a moisturizer.

Make sure to get some fresh air and a little sunshine each day, since these are necessary for healthy skin (and overall good health, too, of course).

Dry skin brushing is highly recommended; see the instructions in chapter 47.

QUICK REVIEW

→ Be careful about what you put on your skin. Chemicals in personal care products are readily absorbed and can harm your body.

→ Opt for nontoxic store-bought or homemade skin care products.

→ Take care of your skin naturally by drinking lots of water; eating fruits, vegetables, and other foods high in antioxidants; turning the heat down in the shower; using coconut oil as a moisturizer; dry brushing your skin; and getting fresh air and a little sunshine every day.

CHOCOLATE MINT SUGAR SCRUB

Makes enough to fill one 12-oz/360-ml jar

This scrub, adapted from the lovely book EcoBeauty (2009) by Lauren Cox with Janice Cox, smells fantastic and works great as a body polisher in the shower. I've used it on my face, too, but if you have really sensitive skin, it might be too abrasive for you (consider mixing in some rolled oats if that's the case).

1 cup/200 g organic or raw sugar

2 tbsp raw cacao or cocoa powder, *preferably fair trade*

¼ or ½ cup/60 to 120 ml almond, avocado, or jojoba oil

1 or 2 drops all-natural peppermint essential oil

1 or 2 drops vitamin E oil *(optional)*

EQUIPMENT

One 12-oz/360-ml glass canning jar with a tight-fitting lid

1 Clean the glass jar and lid in hot, soapy water, or use the hottest setting on your dishwasher.

2 Mix together the sugar and cocoa powder in a medium bowl. Stir in ¼ cup/60 ml of the almond oil. Add more of the oil, 1 tbsp at a time, until your scrub has the desired consistency. Add the essential oil and the vitamin E oil, if desired.

3 Spoon the scrub into the glass jar. It's now ready to use. Store, tightly covered, in a cool place, and it will last for several weeks.

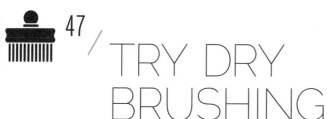

47 / TRY DRY BRUSHING

YOU'VE PROBABLY NEVER HEARD OF DRY BRUSHING YOUR SKIN, but it's a great way to cleanse and stimulate your body's largest eliminative organ. Dry brushing opens the pores, helping to remove dead skin cells. It's also a way to get rid of potentially problematic chemicals that can gather beneath the skin's surface (from soaps, skin creams, deodorants, and antiperspirants, plus synthetic fibers worn next to the skin).

When you dry brush your skin, you also improve your circulation and help your lymphatic system move accumulated toxins out of the lymph glands, which strengthens the function of your immune system. On top of all these unseen benefits, dry skin brushing tightens the skin and can also help to remove cellulite, giving the skin a smoother appearance.

Dry skin brushing is good for anyone who desires skin that looks and feels healthy, and it is specifically recommended when you are doing any type of detox. It can even enhance your digestion!

In order to dry brush your skin properly, you should purchase a loofah or natural-fiber brush with a long handle. These are available at most natural food stores (and online). Plan to do your dry brushing before showering or bathing; it's best if you can do it once a day, but a few times a week is good, too.

Give yourself five to fifteen minutes to brush your whole body. You can start with your feet and move up your body, or you can start high and work your way down. Take care with areas that have thin skin and are generally sensitive, such as the face, breasts, and stomach, and avoid damaged skin or very sensitive areas (I think you know which ones I mean). Use circular motions, brushing toward your heart. On your abdomen, brush in a counterclockwise direction in order to benefit your digestion (simulating the path your food takes as it travels along the digestive process).

After you do your dry brushing, you should take a warm or cold, not hot, shower; at the very least, end with a cold rinse (recall from chapter 46 that this is great for your skin and hair). After you towel off, you can apply some lique-fied organic coconut oil for a skin-softening treat.

QUICK REVIEW

⇥ Dry skin brushing helps remove toxins, improves circulation, and makes your skin feel and look better.

⇥ Purchase a natural-fiber brush and try to do your dry skin brushing every day. Use circular motions, brushing toward your heart, and brushing counterclockwise on your abdomen in order to benefit your digestion.

⇥ Following your dry brushing with a warm or cold, but not hot, shower is best for your skin.

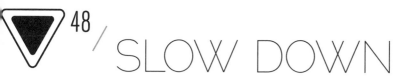

48 / SLOW DOWN

ONCE UPON A TIME (not too long ago), I was obsessed with being productive, with crossing stuff off one checklist or another. My mind was racing all the time with thoughts of everything I needed to do, and I rushed through most tasks just to get them finished.

I used to be afraid to slow down because I feared I would never get anything done. How could I if I didn't rush? Now I understand that by slowing down (and being mindful), I can see clearly what I actually need to do. And if I go at it slowly, I generally do a much better job. *Don't confuse slowing down with procrastinating, though—they are not the same thing.*

I also used to worry that if I slowed down, I'd be late. Now I see that this just isn't the case. Being late is more often about not leaving yourself enough time to prepare. Have you ever had the experience of being in such a rush that you spill your breakfast all over your clothes? Then you need to clean up the mess and go change, and you've wasted a whole bunch of time as a result? I certainly have. I've also gotten a speeding ticket when I was rushing to be somewhere. Of course I ended up late as a result.

Slowing down may require you to adjust your schedule. For example, you may need to start getting up earlier so that you can move at a slower pace in the morning and still get to where you need to be on time. I've personally been getting up half an hour earlier than I used to on weekday mornings so that I don't have to rush through the process of getting my kids ready for school.

Practice taking your time as often as you can. Slow down when you cook, and slow down when you eat; your meals will taste better and you will digest your food better, too. And try to slow down in your interactions with family, friends, and everyone you encounter. If your job lends itself to slowing down, then by all means do so. But definitely slow down when you're at play. Slowing down lets you see things you might have otherwise missed. *Know that slowing down does not equal being lazy; if something is worth doing, it's worth doing slowly.*

For those of us who spend a lot of time online, this may mean reining in an overactive social media existence. I was once on the social media "hamster wheel," but I let it go. It's kind of amazing how much less busy I feel, and how much extra time I've freed up to do other things that are more important to me. I don't know about you, but I have noticed that I experience imagery and information overload when I spend too much time online.

It's good to do an occasional social media "fast." Go away (or stay home) and unplug from the computer and your smartphone for a little while. How long you do this is up to you—it could be five hours or five days. This will allow you to take a break from that pressure to stay connected.

Here are some other tips already covered in this book that can help you slow down:

1. **Close your eyes and take ten very deep, slow breaths in and out. Try this anytime you feel overly busy and stressed.**

2. **Go for a walk or get some other form of exercise.**

3. **Get some fresh air every day and make time to connect with nature.**

4. **Make sure you get enough sleep.**

5. **Schedule downtime into your day to read or do a hobby that you enjoy.**

QUICK REVIEW

⇨ Don't rush through life—it's a marathon, not a sprint.

⇨ Give yourself permission to take it slow sometimes (and to take time off when you need it).

⇨ Slowing down is a good strategy for dealing with anxiety; it's also a good way to help manage stress.

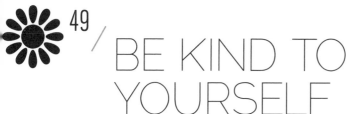

49 / BE KIND TO YOURSELF

I'VE ONLY BEEN AWARE OF THE TERM "SELF-COMPASSION" for a fraction of the fortysomething years that I've been alive. I sure wish I'd learned about it sooner, because I have a history of being quite unkind to myself. Do you have an inner voice that's overly critical, too?

We teach our children to say nice things (or not to say anything at all), and we must teach this to our inner voice, too. We need to have reasonable expectations for ourselves, so we don't set ourselves up for failure. We shouldn't beat ourselves up when things don't go the way we planned; we should pat ourselves on the back when things are going well—and even when they're not. If we were all kinder to ourselves, I think we'd all suffer a lot less, and there would be less need for so many people to be medicated for anxiety and depression.

Being kind to yourself means not judging yourself harshly for not being perfect. It means not holding yourself to impossibly high standards. It means putting an end to comparing yourself to others and to beating yourself up for making a mistake, or for not being good enough at something.

Being kind to yourself means being your own cheerleader. When you are consistently kind to yourself, you don't need others to validate your efforts and boost your self-confidence, because you can do those things for yourself.

I know from personal experience that when your inner monologue regularly engages in overwhelmingly negative banter, this eats away at your self-esteem and keeps you from being truly happy and healthy. Banishing negative self-talk isn't something that can be accomplished in one day, though; it can take time. Here are some steps to take that have worked for me: Surround yourself with encouraging, supportive friends; recite positive affirmations every day (don't knock it until you try it!); learn how to be in the moment; make a conscious effort to choose optimism over pessimism; and practice gratitude (more on this in the next chapter). Like I said, this all takes time. It is a process.

Let's be clear that being kind to yourself does not mean you give yourself permission to spend the day on the couch eating bonbons. Quite the contrary. Being kind to yourself means respecting your body, so that you take excellent care of yourself. Being kind to yourself means you are more likely to eat healthy food, get enough sleep, and exercise regularly. When you are kind to yourself, you'll feel better mentally and physically. You'll be more likely to excel at all that you do, and you'll be better able to take good care of others.

QUICK REVIEW

→ Be kind to yourself! Train your inner voice to say nice things, and to be positive.

→ Don't beat yourself up for not being perfect and don't compare yourself to others. Be your own cheerleader; don't look to others to boost your self-esteem.

→ Be kind to yourself by putting the best quality food into your body, getting enough sleep, and exercising regularly. This will allow you to be the best you that you can be, and to take excellent care of those you love.

THANK YOU!

50 / PRACTICE GRATITUDE

DO YOU SPEND A LOT OF TIME THINKING about what's wrong with your life and what you are lacking? If so, I want to encourage you to start practicing gratitude. I firmly believe we must appreciate everything we have before anything different—and potentially good—can come our way. We must be grateful for the past and the present in order for positive change to be possible in the future.

Life isn't always easy, and bad things do happen, but it's a heck of a lot more pleasant—and it fosters a truly healthy mental state—if you've got an attitude of gratitude. Practicing gratitude can calm you down when you're feeling anxious; it can also help you reverse negative thought patterns (at least it does for me). Practicing gratitude makes you more open to the possibility of positive experiences, and it's a pretty effective way to turn a bad day around. I really can't recommend it enough.

I try to devote some time to thinking about and being thankful for everything good that exists in my life each and every day. What's on my list right now? My family, my friends, a healthy and strong body, my house, my pets, good food on my table, the ability to do work that I love (like writing this book), and the opportunity to connect with others through my blog.

Have there been and are there still negative things in my life? Sure. But guess what? I am thankful for those, too. While there is part of me that wishes I had not wasted all those years obsessing over my weight and dieting my health into the ground, I am honestly grateful for the experience. Without it, I would not have gone on to discover my passion for holistic health and nutrition or been able to share it with others.

Life is so brief—why not share your gratitude? Studies have found that couples who express gratitude to one another have better relationships than those who do not. Tell those who help you out that you appreciate them. Pick up the phone and make a call, or send a thank-you note to let someone know that you are grateful for something they did, or simply that you are glad they are a part of your world.

QUICK REVIEW

→ Adopt an attitude of gratitude. Don't dwell on what your life is lacking: Be thankful for what you already have. Being grateful for the past opens the door for positive change in the future. Spend time practicing gratitude every day, and don't forget to share your gratitude with others.

ACKNOWLEDGMENTS

IN THE SPIRIT OF GRATITUDE, I'd like to take this opportunity to extend a giant "thanks!" to *you*. Thank you for reading what I have to say, both here and on my blog. The process of writing the "One Simple Change" series for Healthy Green Kitchen, and then turning the series into this book, has been a wonderful experience for me. I thank you for being a part of it. I also want to thank my friends and family. Your love and support mean the world to me, and I appreciate you all so much. And a special shout-out of gratitude goes to the following folks (without whom this book would not exist):

Thank you, Kim Foster, for being my sounding board: I adore our daily chats. Thank you, Dianne Jacob, for your wise advice on many occasions, and for reminding me about the power of positive affirmations; thank you, Leigh Haber, for seeing potential in this project before I did; thank you, Jenni Ferrari-Adler, for walking me through my first book experience, and for reassuring me whenever there was a bump in the road; thank you, Lorena Jones, Lisa Tauber, and the team at Chronicle, for making my goal of writing a book a reality.

Thank you, Maddie and Dylan, for always keeping me on my toes, and for teaching me how to be a better person each and every day: You are brilliant, kind, and talented, and I am lucky to be your mom. Thank you, Dan, for being so supportive (and just awesome all around). And last but not least, a giant thank-you to my parents for instilling in me a respect for real food early on, and for encouraging me to follow the beat of my own drum—I love you.

SELECTED BIBLIOGRAPHY

Albala, Ken and Rosanna Nafziger. *The Lost Art of Real Cooking: Rediscovering the Pleasures of Traditional Food One Recipe at a Time*. New York: Perigee, 2010.

Bach, David with Hillary Rosner. *Go Green, Live Rich: 50 Simple Ways to Save the Earth*. New York: Broadway Books, 2008.

Ballard, Tom. *Nutrition-1-2-3: Three Proven Diet Wisdoms for Gaining Energy, Losing Weight and Reversing Chronic Disease*. Seattle, WA: Fresh Press Books, 2008.

Batmanghelidj, F. *Your Body's Many Cries for Water*. Falls Church, VA: Global Health Solutions, 1995.

Bond, Annie B., Melissa Breyer, and Wendy Gordon. *True Food: 8 Simple Steps to a Healthier You*. Washington, DC: National Geographic, 2010.

Braly, James, and Patrick Holford. *Hidden Food Allergies: The Essential Guide to Uncovering Hidden Food Allergies—and Achieving Permanent Relief*. Laguna Beach, CA: Basic Health Publications, 2006.

Calbom, Cherie, and John Calbon. *Sleep Away the Pounds: Optimize Your Sleep and Reset Your Metabolism for Maximum Weight Loss*. New York: Wellness Central, 2007.

Cassity, Jessica. *Better Each Day: 365 Expert Tips for a Healthier, Happier You*. San Francisco: Chronicle Books, 2011.

Chek, Paul. *How to Eat, Move and Be Healthy: Your Personalized 4-step Guide to Looking and Feeling Great from the Inside Out*. San Diego: C.H.E.K Institute, 2004.

Chernila, Alana. *The Homemade Pantry: 101 Foods You Can Stop Buying and Start Making*. New York: Clarkson Potter, 2012.

Cox, Lauren with Janice Cox. *EcoBeauty: Rubs, Masks, and Bath Bombs for You and Your Friends*. Berkeley: Ten Speed Press, 2009.

D'Adamo, Peter with Catherine Whitney. *Eat Right 4 Your Type: The Individualized Diet Solution to Staying Healthy, Living Longer and Achieving Your Ideal Weight*. New York: G.P. Putnam's Sons, 1996.

Davis, William. *Wheat Belly: Lose the Wheat, Lose the Weight, and Find Your Way Back to Health*. New York: Rodale, 2011.

Ehrlich, Richard. *The Green Kitchen: Techniques and Recipes for Cutting Energy Use, Saving Money and Reducing Waste*. London: Kyle Books, 2009.

Enig, Mary. *Know Your Fats: The Complete Primer for Understanding the Nutrition of Fats, Oils, and Cholesterol*. Silver Spring, MD: Bethesda Press, 2000.

Fallon, Sally with Pat Connolly and Mary G. Enig. *Nourishing Traditions: The Cookbook that Challenges Politically Correct Nutrition and the Diet Dictocrats*. San Diego: ProMotion Publishing, 1995.

Goldsmith, Sheherazade, editor-in-chief. *A Slice of Organic Life*. New York: Dorling Kindersley, 2007.

Goodman, Myra. *The Earthbound Cook: 250 Recipes for Delicious Food and a Healthy Planet*. New York: Workman Publishing, 2010.

Graham, Tyler and Drew Ramsey. *The Happiness Diet: A Nutritional Prescription for a Sharp Brain, Balanced Mood, and Lean, Energized Body*. New York: Rodale, 2011.

Hayford, Kelly. *If It's Not Food, Don't Eat It! The No-nonsense Guide to an Eating-for-Health Lifestyle*. Boulder, CO: Delphic Corner Press, 2005.

Holick, Michael F. *The Vitamin D Solution: A 3-Step Strategy to Cure Our Most Common Health Problems*. New York: Plume, 2010.

Junger, Alejandro with Amely Greeven. *Clean: The Revolutionary Program to Restore the Body's Natural Ability to Heal Itself*. New York: HarperOne, 2009.

Keith, Lierre. *The Vegetarian Myth: Food, Justice, and Sustainability*. Crescent City, CA: Flashpoint Press, 2009.

Margel, Douglas. *The Nutrient Dense Eating Plan: Enjoy a Lifetime of Super Health with This Fundamental Guide to Exceptional Foods*. Laguna Beach, FL: Basic Health Publications, 2005.

Mendelson, Anne. *Milk: The Surprising Story of Milk Through the Ages*. New York: Knopf, 2008.

Mercola, Joseph with Kendra Pearsall. *Take Control of Your Health*. Schaumburg, IL: Mercola.com, 2007.

Planck, Nina. *Real Food: What to Eat and Why*. New York and London: Bloomsbury Publishing, 2006.

Prentice, Jessica . *Full Moon Feast: Food and the Hunger for Connection*. White River Junction, VT: Chelsea Green Publishing, 2006.

Price, Weston A. *Nutrition and Physical Degeneration*. La Mesa, CA: Price Pottenger Nutrition Foundation, 2004.

Ravnskov, Uffe. *The Cholesterol Myths: Exposing the Fallacy that Saturated Fat and Cholesterol Cause Heart Disease*. Washington, DC: New Trends Publishing, 2000.

Ross, Julia. *The Diet Cure: The 8-Step Program to Rebalance Your Body Chemistry and End Food Cravings, Weight Problems, and Mood Swings—Now*. New York: Penguin Books, 1999.

Sanfilipo, Diane. *Practical Paleo: A Customized Approach to Health and a Whole-Foods Lifestyle*. Las Vegas: Victory Belt Publishing, Inc., 2012.

Schmid, Ron. *The Untold Story of Milk: Green Pastures, Contented Cows and Raw Dairy Products*. Washington, DC: New Trends Publishing, 2003.

Schwarzbein, Diana. *The Schwarzbein Principle, The Program: Losing Weight the Healthy Way*. Deerfield Beach, FL: Health Communications, 2004.

Smith, Melissa Diane. *Going Against the Grain: How Reducing and Avoiding Grains Can Revitalize Your Health*. New York: Contemporary Books, 2002.

Stec, Laura with Eugene Cordero. *Cool Cuisine: Taking the Bite Out of Global Warming*. Layton, UT: Gibbs Smith, 2008.

Taubes, Gary. *Why We Get Fat: And What to Do About It*. New York: Anchor Books, 2010.

Weed, Susun. *Breast Cancer? Breast Health!* Woodstock, NY: Ash Tree Publishing, 1996.

SELECTED REFERENCES

CHAPTERS 1 TO 5

Boschmann, Michael, et al. "Water Drinking Induces Thermogenesis Through Osmosensitive Mechanisms." *The Journal of Clinical Endocrinology and Metabolism* 92 (August 2007): 3334–3337. doi:10.1210/jc.2006-1438.

Brown, Catriona J, et al. "The Erosive Potential of Flavoured Sparkling Water Drinks." *International Journal of Paediatric Dentistry* 17, no. 2 (March 2007): 86–91. doi: 10.1111/j.1365-263X.2006.00784.x.

Figueiro, Mariana G, et al. "Light Modulates Leptin and Ghrelin in Sleep-Restricted Adults." *International Journal of Endocrinology* 2012 (2012). article ID 530726. doi: 10.1155/2012/530726.

Haus, Erhard L, and MH Smolensky. "Shift Work and Cancer Risk: Potential Mechanistic Roles of Circadian Disruption, Light at Night, and Sleep Deprivation." *Sleep Medicine Reviews* (November 2012). doi: 10.1016/j. smrv.2012.08.003.

Heaney, Robert P, and K Rafferty. "Carbonated Beverages and Urinary Calcium Excretion." *American Journal of Clinical Nutrition* 74, no. 3 (September 2001): 343-7.

Hindmarch, I. "A Naturalistic Investigation of the Effects of Day-long Consumption of Tea, Coffee and Water on Alertness, Sleep Onset and Sleep Quality." *Psychopharmacology* 149, no. 3 (April 2000): 203-16.

Janas-Kozik, M, et al. "Orthorexia—a New Diagnosis?" *Polskie Towarzystwo Psychiatryczne* 46, no. 3 (May–June 2012): 441–50.

Jung, CM, et al. "Acute Effects of Bright Light Exposure on Cortisol Levels." *Journal of Biological Rhythms* 25, no. 3 (June 2010): 208-16. doi: 10.1177/0748730410368413.

Maughan, Ron J, et al. "Caffeine Ingestion and Fluid Balance: a Review." *Journal of Human Nutrition and Dietetics* 16, no. 6 (December 2003 Dec): 411-20.

Mercola, Joseph. "Want a Good Night's Sleep? Then Never Do These Things Before Bed." (October 2, 2010). Accessed August, 2012. http://articles.mercola.com/sites/articles/archive/2010/10/02/secrets-to-a-good-night-sleep.aspx.

Mosby, Terezie T, et al. "Nutrition in Adult and Childhood Cancer: Role of Carcinogens and Anti-carcinogens." *AntiCancer Research* 32, no. 10 (October 2012): 4171-92.

Naidenko, Olga, et al. "Bottled Water Contains Disinfection Byproducts, Fertilizer Residue, and Pain Medication." *Environmental Working Group*. October 2008. http://www.ewg.org/reports/BottledWater/Bottled-Water-Quality-Investigation.

National Toxicology Program. "Bisphenol A (BPA)." August 2010. *National Institute of Environmental Health Sciences*. http://www.niehs.nih.gov/health/assets/docs_a_e/bisphenol_a.pdf.

Rubin, Beverly S. "Bisphenol A: an Endocrine Disruptor with Widespread Exposure and Multiple Effects." *The Journal of Steroid Biochemistry and Molecular Biology* 127, no. 1-2 (October 2011): 27-34.

Tucker Katherine L, et al. "Colas, But Not Other Carbonated Beverages, are Associated with Low Bone Mineral Density in Older Women: The Framingham Osteoporosis Study." *American Journal of Clinical Nutrition* 84, no. 4 (October 2006): 936-42.

Van Cauter, Eve, et al. "Metabolic Consequences of Sleep and Sleep Loss." *Sleep Medicine* 9, Suppl. 1 (September 2008): S23–S28. doi: 10.1016/S1389-9457(08)70013-3.

Wang, Tiange, at al. "Urinary Bisphenol A (BPA) Concentration Associates with Obesity and Insulin Resistance." *The Journal of Clinical Endocrinology & Metabolism* 97, no. 2 (February 2012): E223-7. doi: 10.1210/jc.2011-1989.

CHAPTERS 6 TO 10

Babauta, Leo. "Zen Mind: How To Declutter." (January 28, 2007). Accessed February, 2102. http://zenhabits.net/zen-mind-how-to-declutter.

Dinas PC, et al. "Effects of Exercise and Physical Activity on Depression." *Irish Journal of Medical Sciences* 180, no. 2 (June 2011): 319-25. doi: 10.1007/s11845-010-0633-9.

Goh, Jorming, et al. "Exercise, Physical Activity and Breast Cancer: the Role of Tumor-associated Macrophages." *Exercise Immunology Review* 18 (2012): 158-76.

Grant, William B. "Update on Evidence that Support a Role of Solar Ultraviolet-B Irradiance in Reducing Cancer Risk." *Anti-cancer Agents in Medicinal Chemistry* 13, no. 1 (January 2013): 140-146.

Holick, Michael F. "Evidence-based D-bate on Health Benefits of Vitamin D Revisited." *Dermatoendocrinology* 4, no. 2 (April 2012): 183–190.

———. "Photosynthesis of Vitamin D in the Skin: Effect of Environmental and Life-style Variables." *Federation of American Societies for Experimental Biology* 46, no. 5 (April 1987): 1876-82.

Howlett, Trevor A, et al. "Release of Beta Endorphin and Met-enkephalin During Exercise in Normal Women: Response to Training." *British Medical Journal* (Clinical Research Ed.) no. 288 (June 1984): 1950–1952.

Laskowski, Edward R. "The Role of Exercise in the Treatment of Obesity." *PM & R: the Journal of Injury, Function, and Rehabilitation* 4, no. 11 (November 2012): 840-4. doi: 10.1016/j.pmrj.2012.09.576.

Mercola, Joseph. "Little Sunshine Mistakes That Can Give You Cancer Instead of Vitamin D." (March 26, 2012). Accessed September, 2012. http://articles.mercola.com/sites/articles/archive/2012/03/26/maximizing-vitamin-d-exposure.aspx.

———. "Want to Live Longer? Try Vitamin D." (November 26, 2009). Accessed September, 2012. http://articles.mercola.com/sites/articles/archive/2009/11/26/want-to-live-longer-try-vitamin-d.aspx.

Nabkasorn, C, et al. "Effects of Physical Exercise on Depression, Neuroendocrine Stress Hormones and Physiological Fitness in Adolescent Females with Depressive Symptoms." *European Journal of Public Health* 16 no. 2 (April 2006): 179-84.

O'Keefe, James H, et al. "Organic Fitness: Physical Activity Consistent with Our Hunter-gatherer Heritage." *The Physician and Sportsmedicine* 38, no. 4 (December 2010): 11-8. doi: 10.3810/psm.2010.12.1820.

Reichrath, Jorg. "Skin Cancer Prevention and UV-protection: How to Avoid Vitamin D-deficiency?" *The British Journal of Dermatology* 161, Suppl. 3 (November 2009): 54-60.

Subirats, Bayego E, et al. "Exercise Prescription: Indications, Dosage and Side Effects." *Medicina Clínica* 138, no. 1 (January 2012): 18-24. doi: 10.1016/j.medcli.2010.12.008.

Umpierre, Daniel, et al. "Physical Activity Advice Only or Structured Exercise Training and Association with HbA1c levels in Type 2 Diabetes: a Systematic Review and Meta-analysis." *Journal of the American Medical Association* 305, no. 17 (May 2011): 1790-9. doi:10.1001/jama.2011.576.

Westcott, Wayne L. "Resistance Training is Medicine: Effects of Strength Training on Health." *Current Sports Medicine Reports* 11, no. 4 (July-August 2012): 209-16. doi: 10.1249/JSR.0b013e31825dabb8.

CHAPTERS 11 TO 15

Aller, Erik, et al. "Starches, Sugars and Obesity." *Nutrients* 3, no. 3 (March, 2011): 341–369. doi: 10.3390/nu3030341.

Boris, M, and FS Mandel. "Foods and Additives are Common Causes of the Attention Deficit Hyperactive Disorder in Children." *Annals of Allergy* 72, no. 5 (May, 1994): 462-8.

Carrocio A, et al. "Evidence of Very Delayed Clinical Reactions to Cow's Milk in Cow's Milk-intolerant Patients." *Allergy* 55, no. 5 (June 2000): 574-9.

———. "Non-Celiac Wheat Sensitivity Diagnosed by Double-blind Placebo-controlled Challenge: Exploring a New Clinical Entity." *American Journal of Gastroenterology* 107, no.12 (December 2012): 1898-906; doi: 10.1038/ajg.2012.236.

Collino, Massimo. "High Dietary Fructose Intake: Sweet or Bitter Life?" *World Journal of Diabetes* 2, no. 6 (June 2011): 77-81. doi: 10.4239/wjd.v2.i6.77.

Ford, Rodney P. "The Gluten Syndrome: a Neurological Disease." *Medical Hypotheses* 73, no. 3 (September 2009): 438-40. doi: 10.1016/j.mehy.2009.03.037.

Fortuna, JL. "The Obesity Epidemic and Food Addiction: Clinical Similarities to Drug Dependence." *Journal of Psychoactive Drugs* 44, no. 1 (January-March 2012): 56-63.

————. "Sweet Preference, Sugar Addiction and the Familial History of Alcohol Dependence: Shared Neural Pathways and Genes." *Journal of Psychoactive Drugs* 42, no. 2 (June 2010): 147-51.

Hu FB, et al. "Sugar-sweetened Beverages and Risk of Obesity and Type 2 Diabetes: Epidemiologic Evidence." *Physiology & Behavior* 100, no. 1 (April 2010): 47-54. doi: 10.1016/j.physbeh.2010.01.036.

McGough N, and JH Cummings. "Coeliac Disease: a Diverse Clinical Syndrome Caused by Intolerance of Wheat, Barley and Rye." *Proceedings of the Nutrition Society of India* 64, no. 4 (November 2005): 434-50.

Mullin GE, et al. "Testing for Food Reactions: the Good, the Bad, and the Ugly." *Nutrition in Clinical Practice* 25, no. 2 (April 2010): 192-8.

Pelsser, LM, et al. "Effects of a Restricted Elimination Diet on the Behaviour of Children with Attention-deficit Hyperactivity Disorder (INCA study): a Randomised Controlled Trial." *The Lancet* 377, no. 9764 (February 2011): 494-503. doi: 10.1016/S0140-6736(10)62227-1.

Perrier, C, and B Corthésy. "Gut Permeability and Food Allergies." *Clinical and Experimental Allergy* 41, no. 1 (January 2011): 20-8. doi: 10.1111/j.1365-2222.2010.03639.x.

Pietzak, Michelle. "Celiac Disease, Wheat Allergy, and Gluten Sensitivity: When Gluten Free is Not a Fad." *Journal of Parenteral and Enteral Nutrition* 36, Suppl. 1 (January 2012): 68S-75S. doi: 10.1177/0148607111426276.

Rayssiguier, Y, et al. "High Fructose Consumption Combined with Low Dietary Magnesium Intake May Increase the Incidence of the Metabolic Syndrome by Inducing Inflammation." *Magnesium Research* 19, no. 4 (December 2006): 237-43.

Sanchez, Albert, et al. "Role of Sugars in Human Neutrophilic Phagocytosis." *American Journal of Clinical Nutrition* 26, no. 11 (November 1973): 1180-84.

Sapone, Anna, et al. "Spectrum of Gluten-Related Disorders: Consensus on New Nomenclature and Classification." *BMC Medicine* 10, no. 13 (February 2012). doi: 10.1186/1741-7015-10-13.

Seeley, S. "Diet and Breast Cancer: The Possible Connection with Sugar Consumption." *Medical Hypotheses* 11, no. 3 (July 1983): 319-27.

Shambaugh, P, et al. "Differential Effects of Honey, Sucrose, and Fructose on Blood Sugar Levels." *Journal of Manipulative and Physiological Therapeutics* 13, no. 6 (July-August): 322-5.

Spreadbury, Ian. "Comparison with Ancestral Diets Suggests Dense Acellular Carbohydrates Promote an Inflammatory Microbiota, and May Be the Primary Dietary Cause of Leptin Resistance and Obesity." *Diabetes, Metabolic Syndrome and Obesity: Targets and Therapy* 5 (2012): 175-89. doi: 10.2147/DMSO.S33473.

Tappy, Luc, et al. "Fructose and Metabolic Diseases: New Findings, New Questions." *Nutrition* 26, no. 11-12 (November-December): 1044-9. doi: 10.1016/j.nut.2010.02.014.

CHAPTERS 15 TO 19

Caso, J, et al. "The Effect of Carbohydrate Restriction on Prostate Cancer Tumor Growth in a Castrate Mouse Xenograft Model." *Prostate* (October 2012). doi: 10.1002/pros.22586.

Fallon, Sally, and Mary Enig. "The Long Hollow Tube: A Primer on Digestion." (September 23, 2004). Accessed October, 2012. http://www.westonaprice.org/digestive-disorders/primer-digestive-system.

Jönsson, Tommy, et al. "Beneficial Effects of a Paleolithic Diet on Cardiovascular Risk Factors in Type 2 Diabetes: a Randomized Cross-over Pilot Study. *Cardiovascular Diabetology* 8, no. 35 (2009). doi: 10.1186/1475-2840-8-35.

Kowalski, LM, and J Buiko. "Evaluation of Biological and Clinical Potential of Paleolithic Diet." *Roczniki Państwowego Zakładu Higieny* 63, no. 1 (2012): 9-15.

Leite, JO, et al. "Low-carbohydrate Diet Disrupts the Association Between Insulin Resistance and Weight Gain." *Metabolism* 58, no. 8 (August 2009): 1116-22. doi: 10.1016/j.metabol.2009.04.004.

Martin, Corby, et al. "Change in Food Cravings, Food Preferences, and Appetite During a Low-carbohydrate and Low-fat Diet." *Obesity* 19, no. 10 (October 2011): 1963-70. doi: 10.1038/oby.2011.62.

Melnik, Bodo C, et al. "Over-stimulation of Insulin/IGF-1 Signaling by Western Diet May Promote Diseases of Civilization: Lessons Learnt from Laron Syndrome." *Nutrition & Metabolism* 8, vol. 41 (June 2011). doi: 10.1186/1743-7075-8-41.

Varady, Krista A, and Marc K Hellerstein. "Alternate-day Fasting and Chronic Disease Prevention: a Review of Human and Animal trials." *American Journal of Clinical Nutrition* 86, no. 1 (July 2007): 7-13.

CHAPTERS 20 TO 24

Blesso, CN, et al. "Whole Egg Consumption Improves Lipoprotein Profiles and Insulin Sensitivity to a Greater Extent than Yolk-free Egg Substitute in Individuals with Metabolic Syndrome." *Metabolism* 62, no. 3 (September 2012): 400-10. doi: 10.1016/j.metabol.2012.08.014.

Cordain, L, et al. "The Paradoxical Nature of Hunter-gatherer Diets: Meat-based, yet Non-atherogenic." *European Journal of Clinical Nutrition* 56, Suppl. 1 (March 2002 Mar): S42-52.

Daley, Cynthia A, et al. "A Review of Fatty Acid Profiles and Antioxidant Content in Grass-fed and Grain-fed Beef." *Nutrition Journal* 9, no. 10 (March 2010). doi:10.1186/1475-2891-9-10.

Divi, RL, et al. "Anti-thyroid Isoflavones from Soybean: Isolation, Characterization, and Mechanisms of Action." *Biochemical Pharmacology* 54, no. 10 (November 1997): 1087-96.

Ginter, E. "Vegetarian Diets, Chronic Diseases and Longevity." *Bratislavské Lekárske Listy* 109, no. 10 (2008): 463-6.

Jenkins, David, and Andrea R Josse. "Fish oil and Omega-3 Fatty Acids." *Canadian Medical Association Journal* 178, no. 2 (January 2008): 157-64. doi: 10.1503/cmaj.071754.

Kuipers, RS, et al. "Saturated Fat, Carbohydrates and Cardiovascular Disease." *The Netherlands Journal of Medicine* 69, no. 9 (September 2011): 372-8.

McAfee, AJ, et. al. "Red Meat from Animals Offered a Grass Diet Increases Plasma and Platelet n-3 PUFA in Healthy Consumers." *The British Journal of Nutrition* 105, no. 1 (January 2011): 80-9. doi: 10.1017/S0007114510003090.

Mickleborough, TD, et al. "Effect of Fish Oil-derived Omega-3 Polyunsaturated Fatty Acid Supplementation on Exercise-induced Bronchoconstriction and Immune Function in Athletes." *The Physician and Sportsmedicine* 36, no. 1 (December 2008): 11-7.

Petursson, H, et al. "Is the Use of Cholesterol in Mortality Risk Algorithms in Clinical Guidelines Valid? Ten Years Prospective Data from the Norwegian HUNT 2 Study." *Journal of Evaluation in Clinical Practice* 18, no. 1 (February 2012): 159-168. doi: 10.1111/j.1365-2753.2011.01767.x.

Sinn, Natalie, et al. "Oiling the Brain: a Review of Randomized Controlled Trials of Omega-3 Fatty Acids in Psychopathology Across the Lifespan." *Nutrients* 2, no. 2 (February 2010): 128-170. doi: 10.3390/nu2020128.

Siri-Tarino, Patty W, et al. "Meta-analysis of Prospective Cohort Studies Evaluating the Association of Saturated Fat with Cardiovascular Disease." *American Journal of Clinical Nutrition* 91, no. 3 (March 2010): 535-46. doi: 10.3945/ajcn.2009.27725.

———. "Saturated fat, Carbohydrate, and Cardiovascular Disease." *American Journal of Clinical Nutrition* 91, no. 3 (March 2010): 502-9. doi: 10.3945/ajcn.2008.26285.

Werkö, Lars. "End of the Road for the Diet-heart Theory?" *Scandinavian Cardiovascular Journal* 42, no 4 (August 2008): 250-5.

Wertz, PW. "Essential Fatty Acids and Dietary Stress." *Toxicology and Industrial Health* 25, no. 4-5 (May-June 2009): 279-83.

CHAPTERS 26 TO 30

Divi, RL, et al. "Anti-thyroid Isoflavones from Soybean: Isolation, Characterization, and Mechanisms of Action." *Biochemical Pharmacology* 54, no. 10 (November 1997): 1087-96.

Djoussé, Luc, et al. "Chocolate Consumption is Inversely Associated with Prevalent Coronary Heart Disease: the National Heart, Lung, and Blood Institute Family Heart Study." *Clinical Nutrition* 30, no. 2 (April 2011): 182-7. doi: 10.1016/j.clnu.2010.08.005.

Doerge, DR, and Sheehan DM. "Goitrogenic and Estrogenic Activity of Soy Isoflavones." *Environmental Health Perspective* 110, Suppl. 3 (June 2002): 349-53.

Dunne, C, et al. "Probiotics: from Myth to Reality. Demonstration of Functionality in Animal Models of Disease and in Human Clinical Trials." *Antonie Van Leeuwenhoek* 76, no. 1-4 (July-November 1999): 279-92. Heinrich Ulrike, et al. "Long-term Ingestion of High Flavanol Cocoa

Provides Photoprotection Against UV-induced Erythema and Improves Skin Condition in Women." *The Journal of Nutrition* 136, no. 6 (June 2006): 1565-9.

Grassi, Davide, et al. "Short-term Administration of Dark Chocolate is Followed by a Significant Increase in Insulin Sensitivity and a Decrease in Blood Pressure in Healthy Persons." *The American Journal of Clinical Nutrition* 81, no. 3 (March 2005): 611-614.

Jefferson, Wendy N. "Adult Ovarian Function Can Be Affected by High Levels of Soy." *Journal of Nutrition* 140, no. 12 (December 2010): 2322S-2325S. doi: 10.3945/jn.110.123802.

Messina, Mark, et al. "Effects of Soy Protein and Soybean Isoflavones on Thyroid Function in Healthy Adults and Hypothyroid Patients: a Review of the Relevant Literature." *Thyroid* 16, no. 3 (March 2006): 249-58.

Morrell, Sally Fallon. "The Great Iodine Debate." (June 22, 2009). Accessed November, 2012. http://www.westona price.org/metabolic-disorders/the-great-iodine-debate.

Planells E, et al. "Ability of a Cocoa Product to Correct Chronic Mg Deficiency in Rats." *International Journal for Vitamin and Nutrition Research* 69, no. 1 (January 1999): 52-60.

Smyth, Peter PA. "The Thyroid, Iodine and Breast Cancer." *Breast Cancer Research* 5, no. 5 (2003): 235-8.

CHAPTERS 31 TO 35

Bernstein Adam M, et al. "Soda Consumption and the Risk of Stroke in Men and Women." *American Journal of Clinical Nutrition* 95, no. 5 (May 2012): 1190-9. doi: 10.3945/ajcn.111.030205.

Bradley, Patrick. "Diet Composition and Obesity." *The Lancet* 379, no. 9821 (March 2012): 1100. doi:10.1016/S0140-6736(12)60455-3.

Carroccio, A, et al. "Evidence of Very Delayed Clinical Reactions to Cow's Milk in Cow's Milk-intolerant Patients." *Allergy* 55, no. 6 (June 2000): 574-9. doi: 10.1034/j.1398-9995.2000.00417.x.

Fung Teresa T, et al. "Sweetened Beverage Consumption and Risk of Coronary Heart Disease in Women." *American Journal of Clinical Nutrition* 89, no. 4 (April 2009):1037-42. doi: 10.3945/ajcn.2008.27140.

Heaney, Robert P, and Karen Rafferty. "Carbonated Beverages and Urinary Calcium Excretion." *American Journal of Clinical Nutrition* 74, no. 3 (September 2001): 343-7.

Hu, Frank B, and Vasanti S Malik. "Sugar-sweetened Beverages and Risk of Obesity and Type 2 Diabetes: Epidemiologic Evidence." *Physiology & Behavior* 100, no. 1 (April 2010): 47-54. doi: 10.1016/j.physbeh.2010.01.03.

Malik, Vasanti S, et al. "Sugar-sweetened Beverages and Risk of Metabolic Syndrome and Type 2 Diabetes: a Meta-analysis." *Diabetes Care* 33, no. 11 (November 2010): 2477-83. doi: 10.2337/dc10-1079.

Patil, Harshal, et al. "Cuppa Joe: Friend or Foe? Effects of Chronic Coffee Consumption on Cardiovascular and Brain Health." *Missouri Medicine* 108, no. 6 (November-December 2011): 431-8.

Schernhammer, Eva S, et al. "Consumption of Artificial Sweetener- and Sugar-containing Soda and Risk of Lymphoma and Leukemia in Men and Women." *American Journal of Clinical Nutrition* 96, no. 6 (December 2012): 1419-1428. doi: 10.3945/ajcn.111.030833.

Tandel, Kirtida R. "Sugar Substitutes: Health Controversy Over Perceived Benefits." *The Journal of Pharmacology & Pharmacotherapeutics* 2, no 4 (October-December 2011): 236–243. doi: 10.4103/0976-500X.85936.

Tucker, Katherine L, et al. "Colas, But Not Other Carbonated Beverages, are Associated with Low Bone Mineral Density in Older Women: The Framingham Osteoporosis Study." *American Journal of Clinical Nutrition* 84, no 4 (October 2006): 936-42.

Van Neerven, RJ Joost, et al. "Which Factors in Raw Cow's Milk Contribute to Protection Against Allergies?" *Allergy and Clinical Immunology* 180, no. 4 (October 2012): 853-8. doi: 10.1016/j.jaci.2012.06.050.

Vartanian, Lenny R, et al. "Effects of Soft Drink Consumption on Nutrition and Health: a Systematic Review and Meta-analysis." *American Journal of Public Health* 97, no. 4 (April 2007): 667-75.

Yang, Qing. "Gain Weight by "Going Diet?" Artificial Sweeteners and the Neurobiology of Sugar Cravings." *Yale Journal of Biological Medicine* 83, no. 2 (June 2010): 101–108.

Winkelmayer, Wolfgang C, et al. "Habitual Caffeine Intake and the Risk of Hypertension in Women." *Journal of the American Medical Association* 294, no. 18 (November 2005): 2330-5. doi:10.1001/jama.294.18.2330.

CHAPTERS 36 TO 40

Babauta, Leo. "5 Inspirations for Being in the Moment." (July 12, 2007). Accessed March, 2012. http://zenhabits.net/5-inspirations-for-being-in-the-moment.

Liu, C, et al. "Epidemiological and Experimental Links Between Air Pollution and Type 2 Diabetes." *Toxicologic Pathology* (October 2012).

Söderström M, et al. "The Quality of the Outdoor Environment Influences Childrens Health – a Cross-sectional Study of Preschools." *Acta Paediatrica* (2012). doi: 10.1111/apa.12047.

Talbot, JF, et al. "The Benefits of Nearby Nature for Elderly Apartment Residents." *International Journal of Aging and Human Development* 33, no. 2 (1991): 119-30.

CHAPTERS 41 TO 45

"Final Report on Carcinogens Background Document for Formaldehyde." *National Toxicology Program* (January 22, 2010). Accessed December, 2012. http://ntp.niehs.nih.gov/ntp/roc/twelfth/2009/November/Formaldehyde_BD_Final.pdf.

"Fungicide Used on Farm Crops Linked to Insulin Resistance." *ScienceDaily* (June 25, 2012). Accessed November 8, 2012. http://www.sciencedaily.com/releases/2012/06/120625100902.htm.

Gül, Süleyman, et al. "Cytotoxic and Genotoxic Effects of Sodium Hypochlorite on Human Peripheral Lymphocytes in Vitro." *Cytotechnology* 59, no 2 (March 2009): 113-9. doi: 10.1007/s10616-009-9201-4.

"Hazardous Substance Fact Sheet: Sodium Hypochlorite." Accessed December, 2012. http://nj.gov/health/eoh/rtkweb/documents/fs/1707.pdf.

"What Is Permaculture?" Accessed December, 2012. http://www.permaculture.co.uk/what-is-permaculture.

CHAPTERS 46 TO 50

Babauta, Leo. "Why Living a Life of Gratitude Can Make You Happy." (September 13, 2007). Accessed May, 2012. http://zenhabits.net/why-living-a-life-of-gratitude-can-make-you-happy.

Barrett, Julia R. "Chemical Exposures: The Ugly Side of Beauty Products." *Environmental Health Perspectives* 113, no. 1 (January 2005): A24.

Crinnion, Walter J. "Toxic Effects of the Easily Avoidable Phthalates and Parabens." *Alternative Medicine Review* 15, no. 3 (September 2010): 190-6.

Gordon, Amie M, et al. "To Have and To Hold: Gratitude Promotes Relationship Maintenance in Intimate Bonds." *The Journal of Personality and Social Psychology* 103, no. 2 (August 2012): 257-74. doi: 10.1037/a0028723.

Harling, Melanie, et al. "Bladder Cancer Among Hairdressers: a Meta-analysis." *Occupational and Environmental Medicine* 67, no. 5 (May 2010): 351-8. doi:10.1136/oem.2009.050195.

Hepp, Nancy M. "Determination of Total Lead in 400 Lipsticks on the U.S. Market Using a Validated Microwave-assisted Digestion, Inductively Coupled Plasma-mass Spectrometric Method." *Journal of Cosmetic Science* 63, no. 3 (May-June 2012): 159-76.

Mercola, Joseph. "Never Put This On Your Skin". Accessed December, 2012. http://www.mercolahealthyskin.com.

Ruldel, Ruthann A, and Laura J Perovich. "Endocrine Disrupting Chemicals in Indoor and Outdoor Air." *Atmospheric Environment* 43, no. 1 (January 2009): 170–181. doi: 10.1016/j.atmosenv.2008.09.025.

Takkouche, Bahi, et al. "Personal Use of Hair Dyes and Risk of Cancer: a Meta-analysis." *Journal of the American Medical Association* 293, no. 20 (May 2005): 2516-25. doi:10.1001/jama.293.20.2516.

Vetenskapsrådet (The Swedish Research Council). "Skin Creams Can Make Skin Drier." *ScienceDaily* (October 23, 2008). Accessed November 24, 2012. http://www.sciencedaily.com/releases/2008/10/081022101500.htm.

U.S Department of Health and Human Services. "What Ingredients are Prohibited from Use in Cosmetics?" (April 27, 2012). Accessed December, 2012. http://www.fda.gov/Cosmetics/ResourcesForYou/Consumers/CosmeticsQA/ucm167234.htm.

INDEX